Ein Buch aus der

BÜCHER MIT HERZ

So geht's mir gut!

BETTINA KIPPER

Reihe

WWW.SOGEHTSMIRGUT.DE

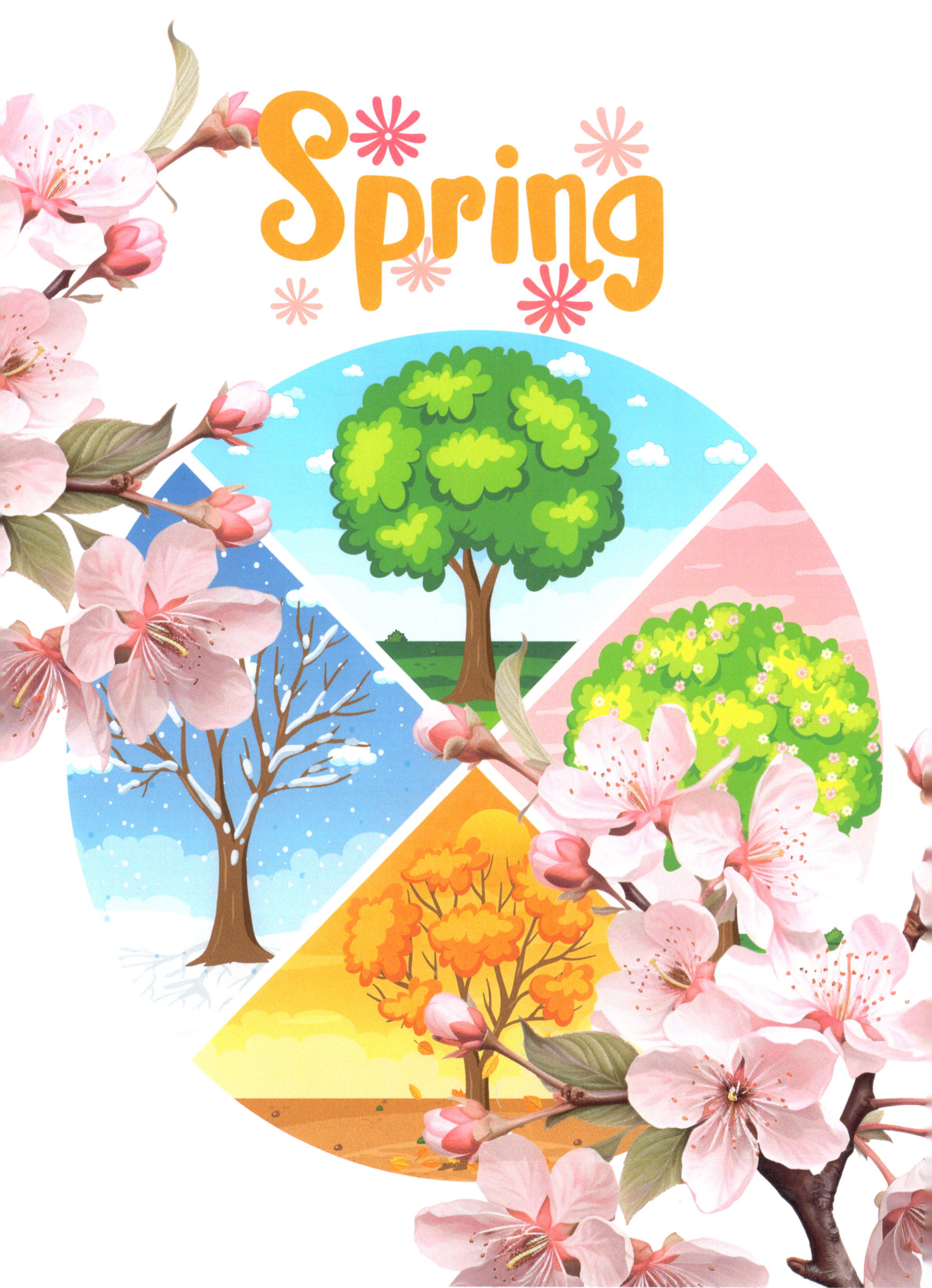

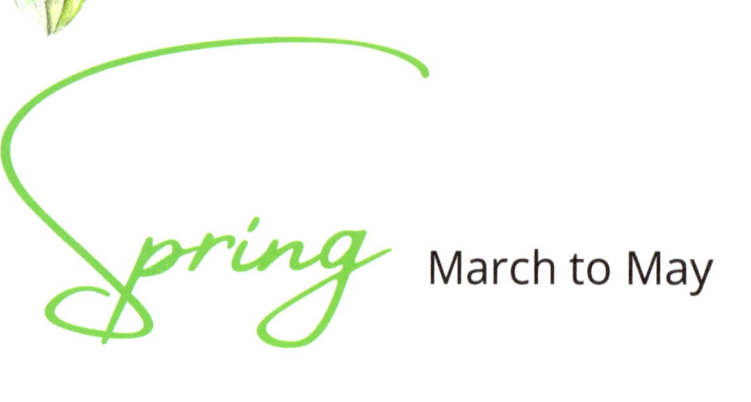 **March to May**

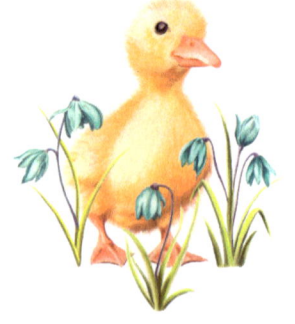

Spring directly follows in the footsteps of winter. In temperate latitudes, nature begins to bloom and everything around us begins to grow.

The length of the day and the arc of the sun change throughout the year, depending on the latitude of a location.

In the Northern Hemisphere, spring begins with the equinox (March 20/21), while in the Southern Hemisphere, autumn begins. Spring in the Southern Hemisphere is different from that in the Northern Hemisphere.

Astronomically speaking, spring ends with the summer solstice (June 20/21), and in the Northern Hemisphere, Meteorologists say spring begins in early March.

In spring we have public holidays such as 1st May. Easter also falls in spring.
Spring pampers us with the first warm rays of sunshine after the long winter. The flowers are starting to bloom, nature is waking up and the days are getting longer again.
Enjoy spring with all its facets.

Yours Bettina Kipper

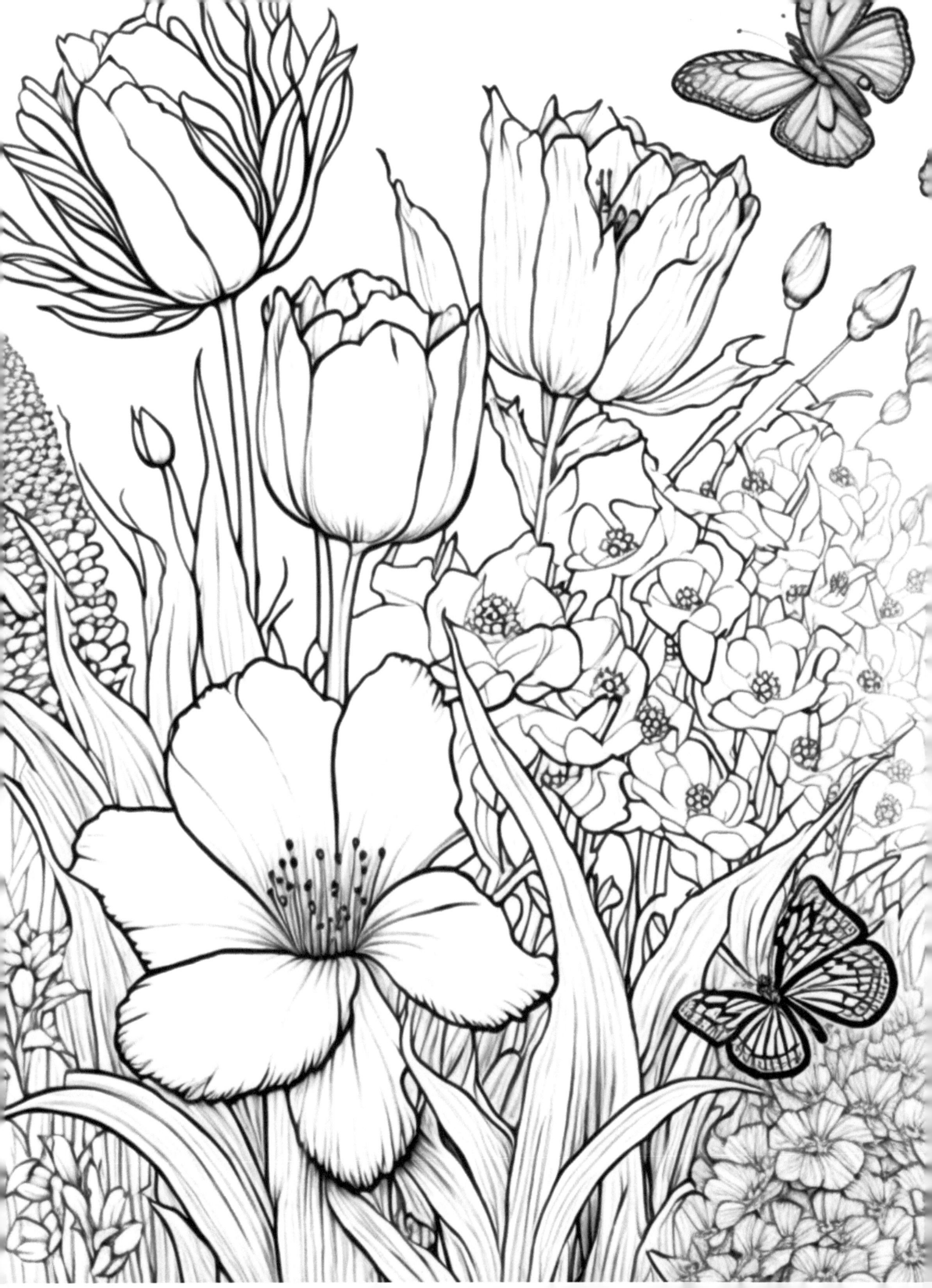

Daisy Bell (1892)

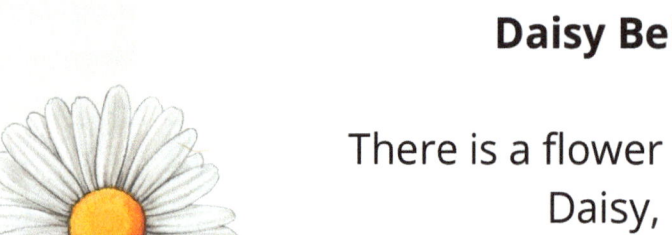
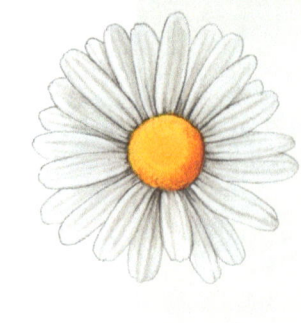

There is a flower within my heart
Daisy, Daisy
Planted one day by a glancing dart
Planted by Daisy Bell
Whether she loves me or loves me not
Sometimes it's hard to tell
Yet I am longing to share the lot
Of beautiful Daisy Bell

Daisy, Daisy, give me your answer, do,
I'm half crazy all for the love of you.
It won't be a stylish marraige
I can't afford the carriage
But you'd look sweet, on the seat
Of a bicycle built for two

We will go tandem as man and wife
Daisy, Daisy
Peddling our way down the road of life
I and my Daisy Bell

When the roads dark and we both dispise
P'licemen and lamps as well.
There are bright lights in the dazzling eyes
Of beautiful Daisy Bell.

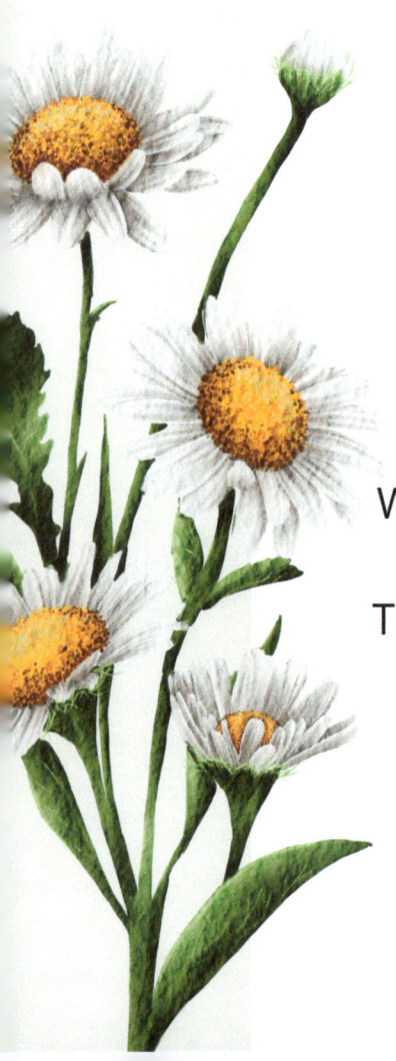

Daisy, Daisy, give me your answer, do,
I'm half crazy all for the love of you.
It won't be a stylish marraige
I can't afford the carriage
But you'd look sweet on the seat
Of a bicycle built for two

I will stand by you in wheel or woe
Daisy, Daisy,
You'll be the bell which I'll ring you know
Sweet little Daisy Bell
You'll take the lead on each trip we take
Then if I don't do well
I will permit you to use the brake
Beautiful Daisy Bell

Daisy, Daisy, give me your answer, do,
I'm half crazy all for the love of you.
It won't be a stylish marraige
I can't afford the carriage
But you'd look sweet on the seat
Of a bicycle built for two

But you'd look sweet on the seat
Of a bicycle built for two
Of a bicycle built for two
Of a bicycle built for two
For two, For two, For two, For two

Harry Dacre 1892

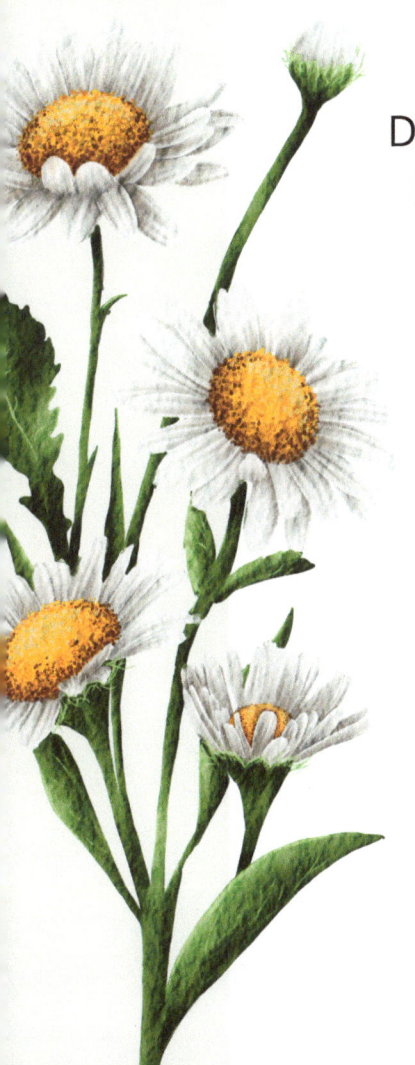

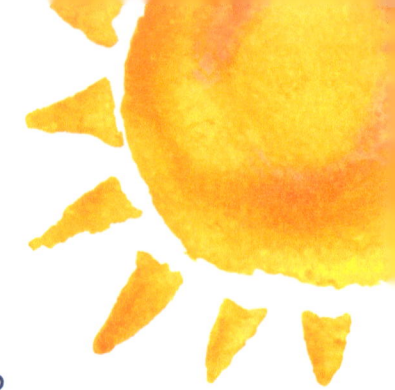

Mirror Mirror:

Can you read the mirrored writing?
We are looking for spring terms

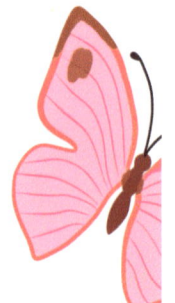

TULIPS

SNOWDROP

DAFFODILS

BUTTERFLY

NARCISSUS

PRIMROSES

BLOOMING

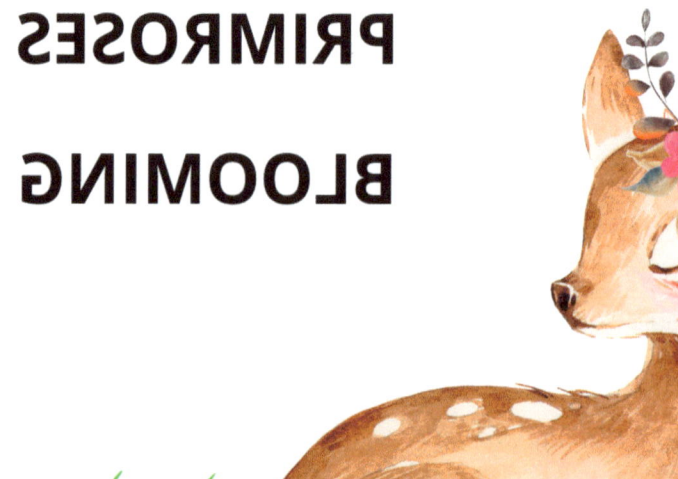

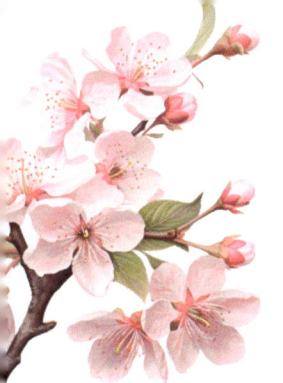
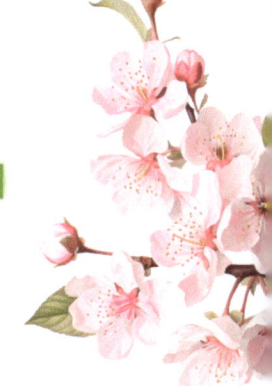

THERE ARE THREE PROVERBS HIDDEN HERE

ONE   A   THE   GRASS

THE   DOES   THE   FLOWERS

WATCHING   MAY   GROW

LIKE   SWALLOW   BRING

MAKE   SHOWERS   NOT

APRIL   THE   SUMMER

April showers bring May flowers.
Like watching grass grow.
One swallow does not make a summer.

↔

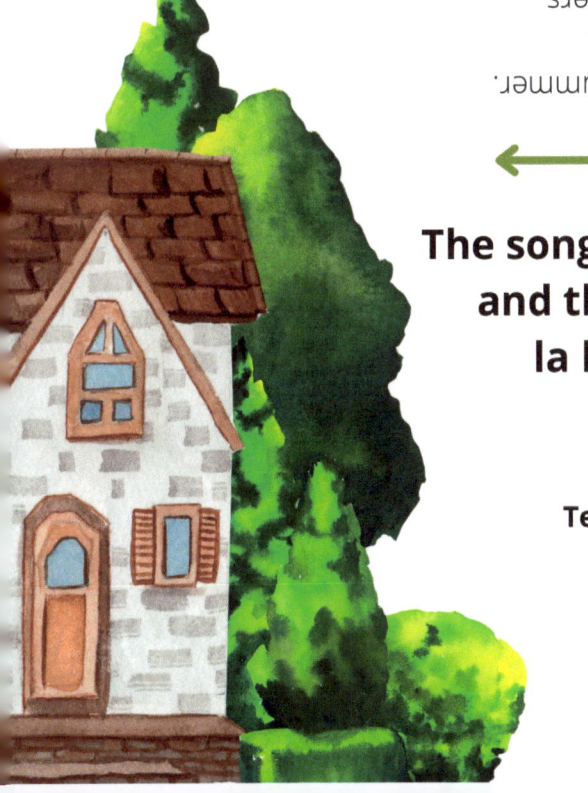

The songs of spring are returning and the shepherd is playing la la la on his shawm...

Text and music: anonymous – from the 19th century

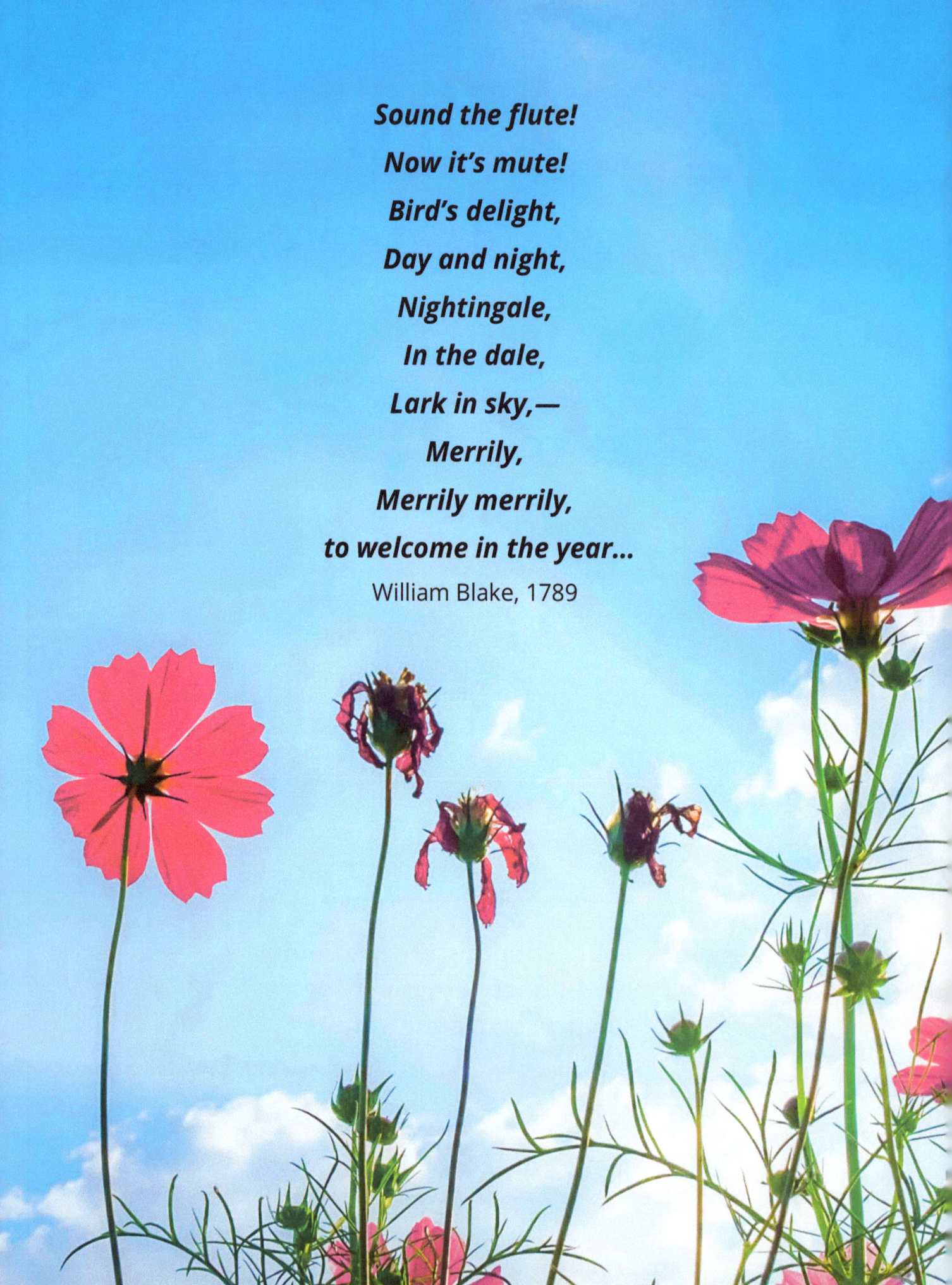

Sound the flute!
Now it's mute!
Bird's delight,
Day and night,
Nightingale,
In the dale,
Lark in sky,—
Merrily,
Merrily merrily,
to welcome in the year...

William Blake, 1789

Separate the endless words into single words in the correct places. The syllables arranged correctly make 11 words about spring.

DRFLOWERSNFODAISYKFT

ULIPJFUTGARDENJFRBIRD

SKFRDSPRINGSJDPLANTIN

GHDKRSUNSHINEKFRTWAR

MKDEASTERKVJUAPRILJD

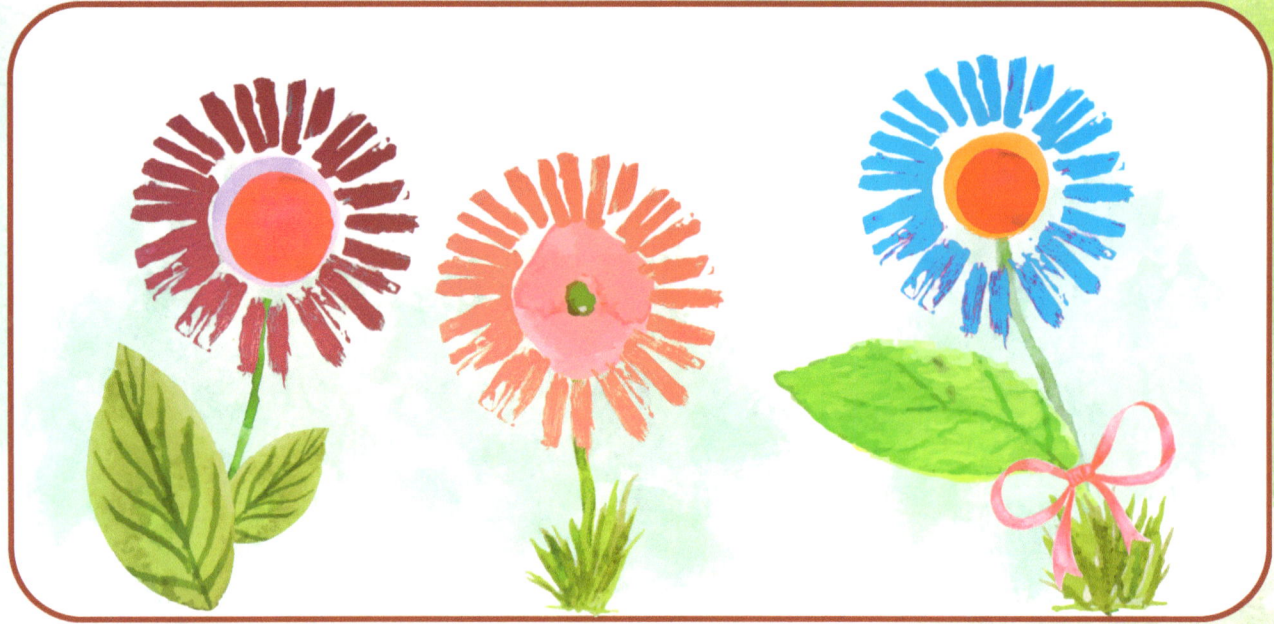

1

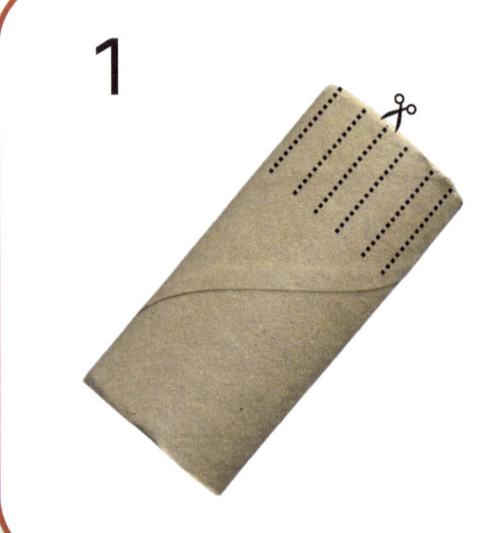

2

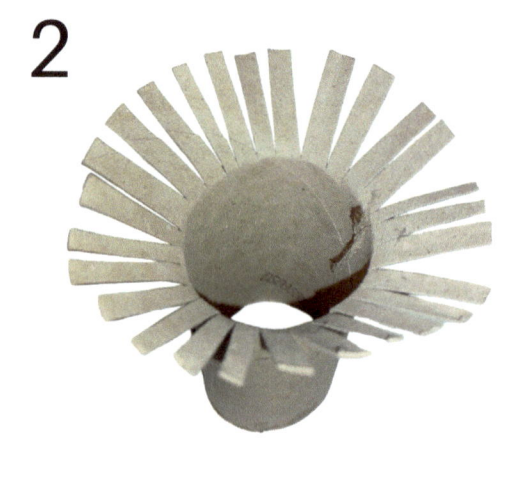

3

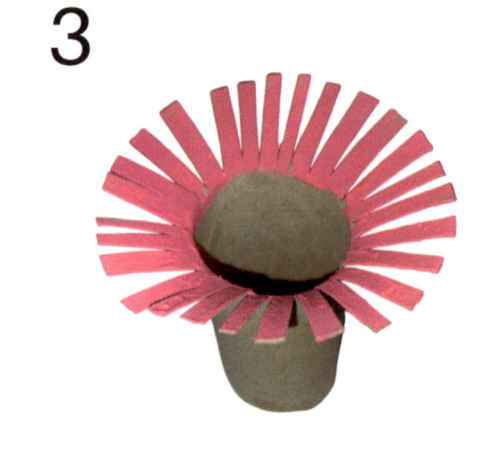

4

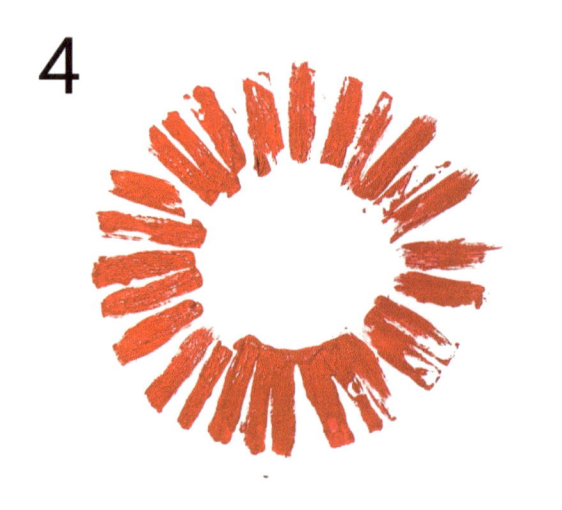

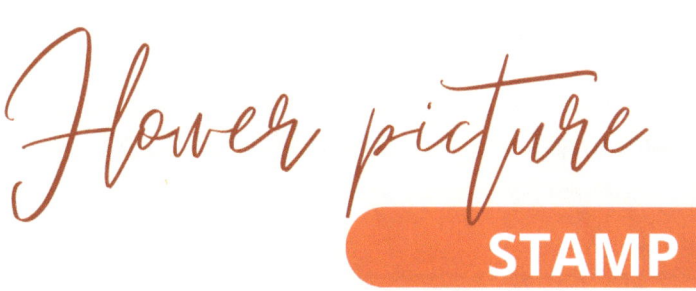

Flower picture

STAMP

You need:

- EMPTY TOILET PAPER ROLLS
- WATERCOLORS OR ACRYLIC PAINTS
- PAINT BRUSH
- PAPER

Here's how it's done:

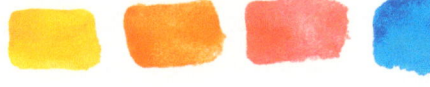

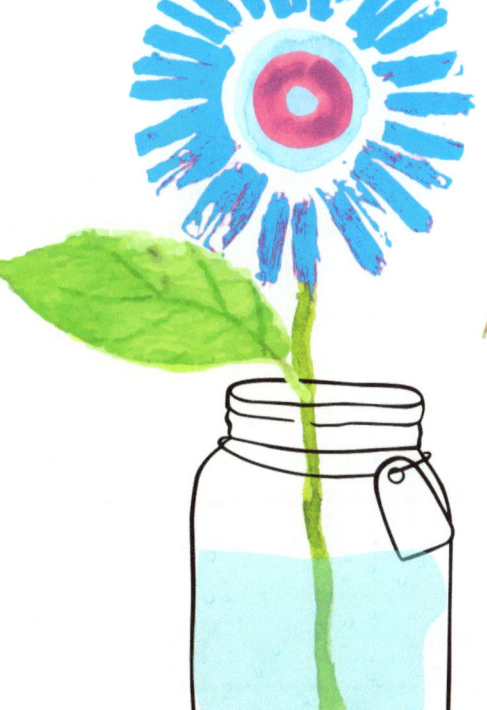

1. Cut the toilet roll with scissors
2. Bend the cut strips outwards
3. Apply paint (watercolor or acrylic paint)
4. Turn the toilet roll over and press the colored side onto the paper.

Now decorate your flowers, give them a few leaves, a stem or put them in a vase.

Spring WORD SEARCH

F	L	C	H	B	C	T	T	S	T	B	A	R	H
F	L	O	W	E	R	S	T	S	P	R	I	N	G
T	O	L	L	E	O	U	L	G	W	G	D	L	R
U	N	O	M	S	C	N	N	R	A	M	C	L	L
L	N	R	A	B	U	T	T	E	R	F	L	Y	I
I	I	S	Y	O	S	C	R	E	M	N	O	N	G
P	N	Ä	X	K	S	N	E	N	T	V	V	M	H
S	S	R	I	B	E	T	I	T	H	R	E	A	T
F	B	L	O	S	S	O	M	S	P	T	T	R	H
P	I	S	U	N	S	H	I	N	E	S	C	C	T
F	A	A	P	R	I	L	C	N	N	N	N	H	M

- FLOWERS
- BUTTERFLY
- SUN
- BEES
- CROCUSSES
- TULIPS
- BLOSSOMS
- GREEN
- COLORS
- WARMTH
- SUNSHINE
- LIGHT
- SPRING
- CLOVE
- APRIL
- MAY
- MARCH

TRIVIA

Test your EASTER knowledge. Most correct answer wins!

1. What color was the first Easter eggs dyed?
   A. Blue   B. Yellow   C. Red

2. What flower is considered an Easter symbol?
   A. Lily   B. Tulip   C. Daisy

3. Easter is commemorated as the day that Jesus was:
   A. Born   B. Resurrected   C. Baptized

4. Where is the largest Easter egg museum in the world?
   A. Germany   B. Ukraine   C. Sweden

5. What country did the Easter Bunny tradition originate?
   A. Germany   B. Poland   C. France

6. What do white Easter Lilies represent?
   A. Optimism   B. wisdom   C. Purity

7. What is the date of Easter determined by?
   A. Weather   B. The moon   C. Date of the month

8. What egg-shaped candy is illegal in the United States?
   A. Cadbury   B. Kinder surprise   C. Robin eggs

9. What kind of meat is often associated with Easter?
   A. Lamb   B. Turkey   C. Pork

10. The most popular American Easter candy is:
    A. Peeps   B. Jelly Beans   C. Cadbury egg

WORD MAZE

Five terms are hidden in this word grid. Find your way through the grid to find the terms. You can only walk vertically and horizontally, not diagonally.

G	D	E	L	O	W
A	R	N	F	R	E
P	W	A	E	R	O
R	O	D	M	E	S
I	O	S	P	R	G
M	R	E	S	I	N

SPRING PROVERBS

A good year is determined by its spring.
(Portugese Proverb)

I love spring anywhere,
but if I could choose
I would always greet it in a garden
Ruth Stout

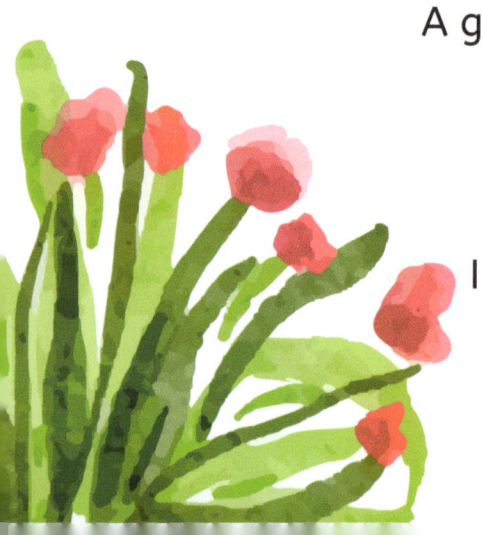

Spring ABC

Can you think of something about spring for each letter in the alphabet?

4

A	_____	M	_____
B	_____	N	_____
C	_____	O	_____
D	_____	P	_____
E	_____	Q	_____
F	_____	R	_____
G	_____	S	_____
H	_____	T	_____
I	_____	U	_____
J	_____	V	_____
K	_____	W	_____
L	_____	X/Y/Z	_____

ABC GAME

At the beginning, decide on a topic, for example spring.
Start on any letter. Then roll the dice and draw the number shown.
Find a term for the selected topic that begins with the letter you landed on.
Keep rolling the dice in turn until no one can think of anything else.
How many terms can you create?

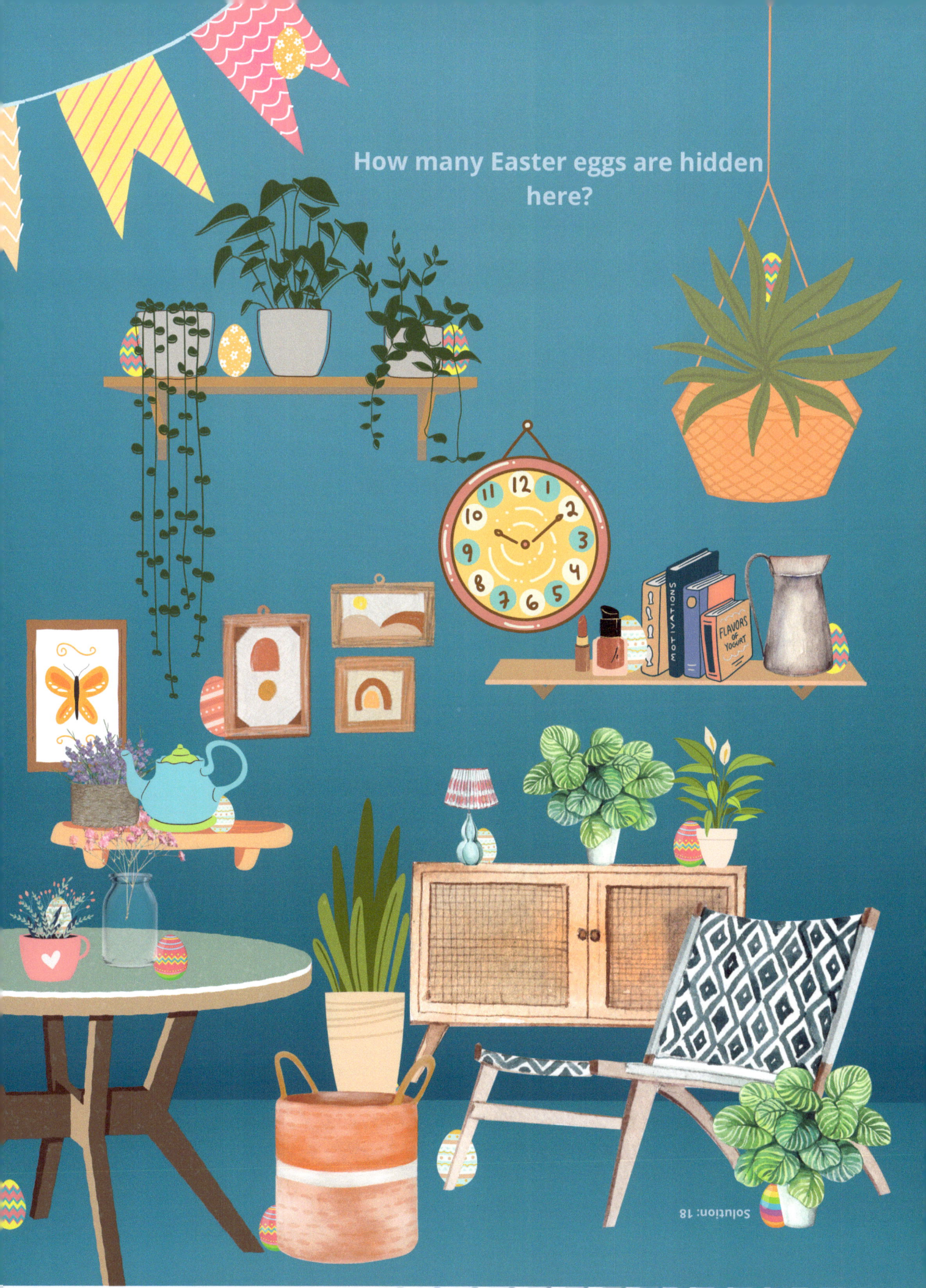

How many Easter eggs are hidden here?

Solution: 18

Daffodils

William Wordsworth

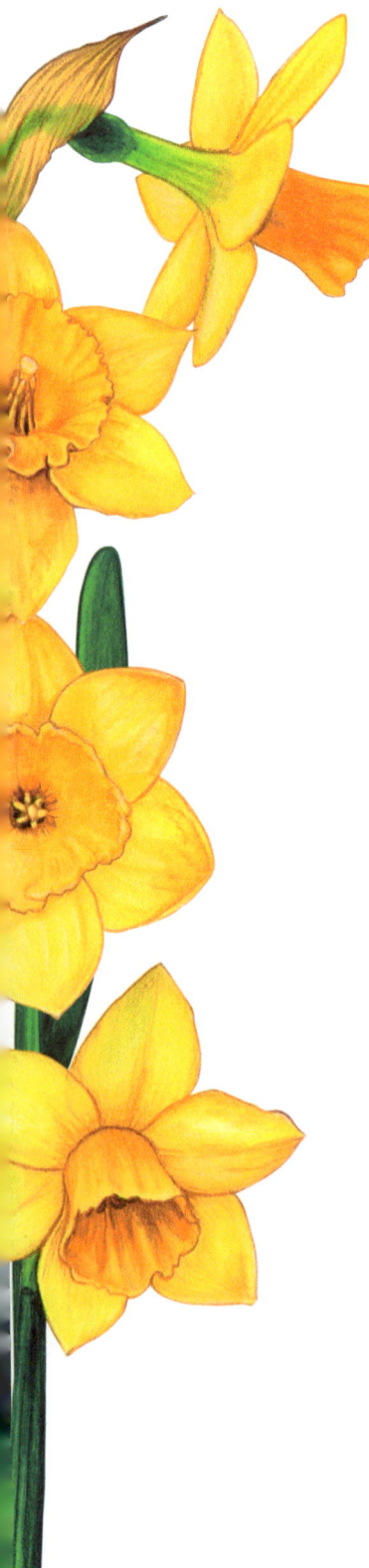

I wandered lonely as a cloud
That floats on high o'er vales and hills,
When all at once I saw a crowd,
A host, of golden daffodils;
Beside the lake, beneath the trees,
Fluttering and dancing in the breeze.

Continuous as the stars that shine
And twinkle on the milky way,
They stretched in never-ending line
Along the margin of a bay:
Ten thousand saw I at a glance,
Tossing their heads in sprightly dance.

The waves beside them danced; but they
Out-did the sparkling waves in glee:
A poet could not but be gay,
In such a jocund company:
I gazed – and gazed – but little thought
What wealth the show to me had brought:

For oft, when on my couch I lie
In vacant or in pensive mood,
They flash upon that inward eye
Which is the bliss of solitude;
And then my heart with pleasure fills,
And dances with the daffodils.

Wordsearch

```
N M L T K I H C C Y W K P M M
G E U L L Z P T T K T N H D B
G N W L T Z S P M H D L B O W
U I M B C R M S T R B U F E Y
A A C Q H Z F U O N A T X Z X
U R G M R B X N E L W B Q K
X Y G H E J P E V P P L F B C
U P E S B K R G B M V X K R M
D B R E I G Z M C X E G D P O
X L S R R B P J U T L D H S S
C O C F T L T S V H E U I V S
A O H T H T A A P W L T H O O
S M W L N K B E O U T X K O L
D X U A H P I C Q E G Y G K B
N K J M Z V P V H J D X V P U
```

1. REBIRTH 2. SUN 3. WARMTH 4. FRESH
5. RAIN 6. BLOOM 7. GREEN 8. BLOSSOM

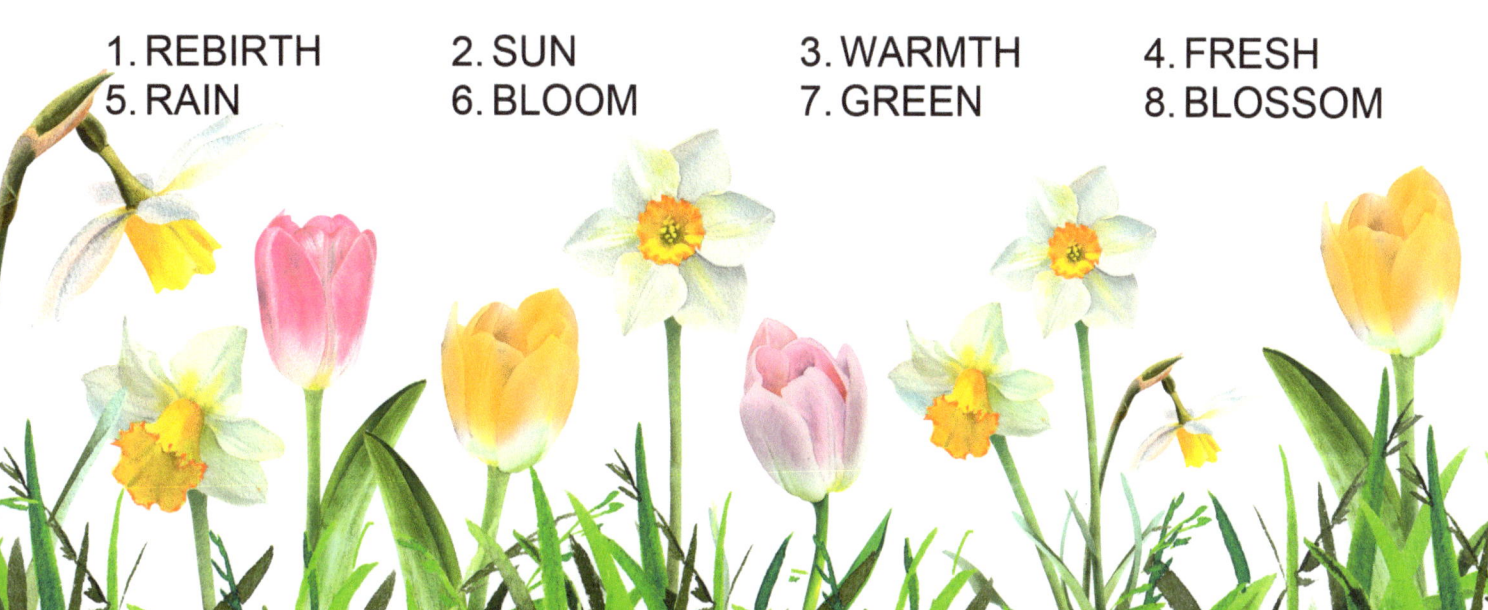

When it becomes warmer..

...it's time to take care of the garden

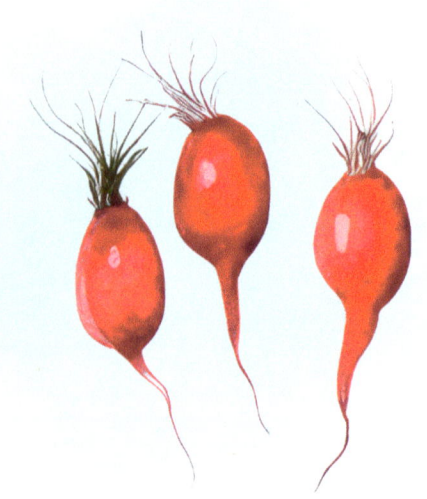

... Radishes can be sown directly in the soil as early as March

... Beetroot can be sown in April and makes a great addition to many dishes.

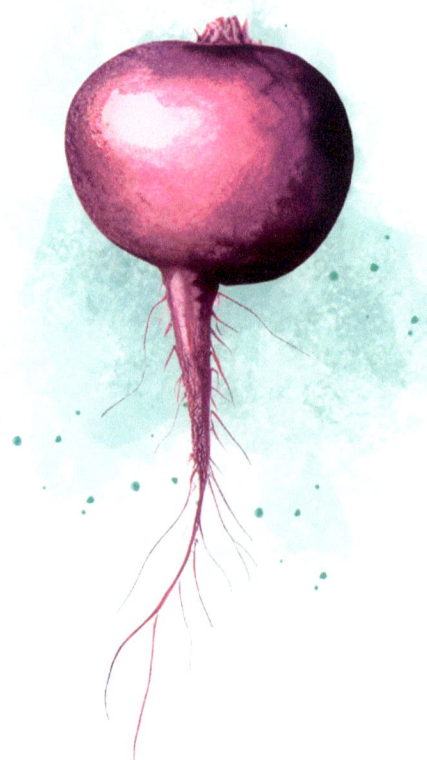

... Lettuce can also be sown in March or April.

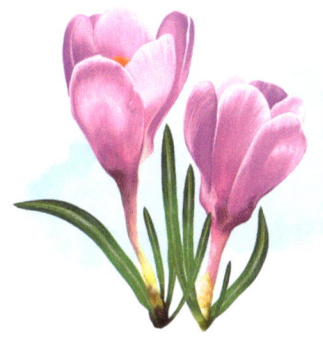

... the spring flowers are starting to bloom, for example the crocuses.

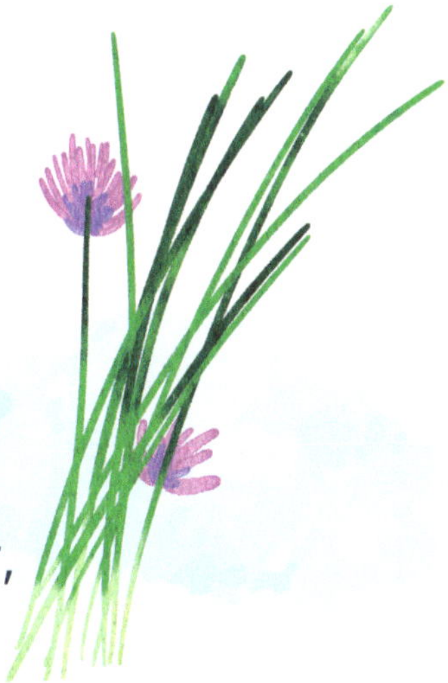

Herbs that have overwintered, such as chives, also come back.

Now it's time to sow, weed, and water, because:

A beautiful garden wipes the dust of everyday life from your soul.

Biographical conversation impulses

What flowers did you have in your garden?

Have you planted herbs and vegetables?

Was gardening fun or was it tiring?

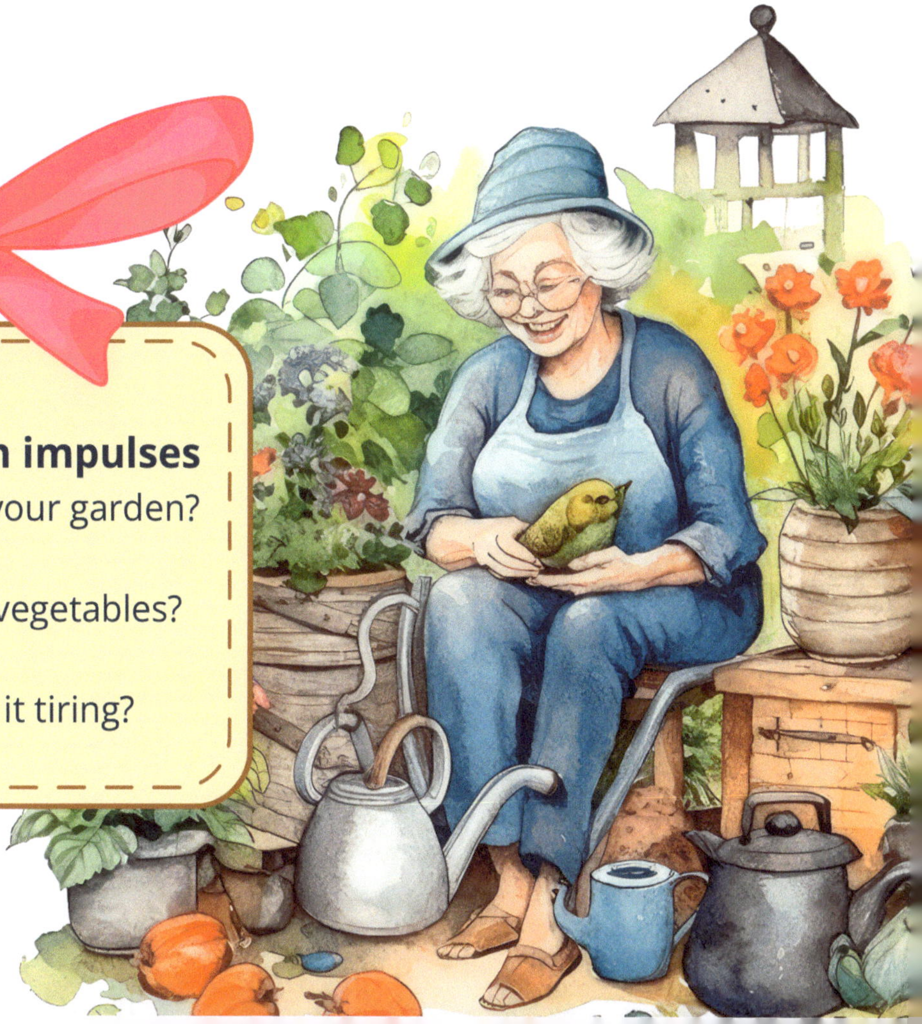

6

How many words can you find in the word

FLOWER MEADOW

TIP: Word searches are also a good way to train memory in a group.

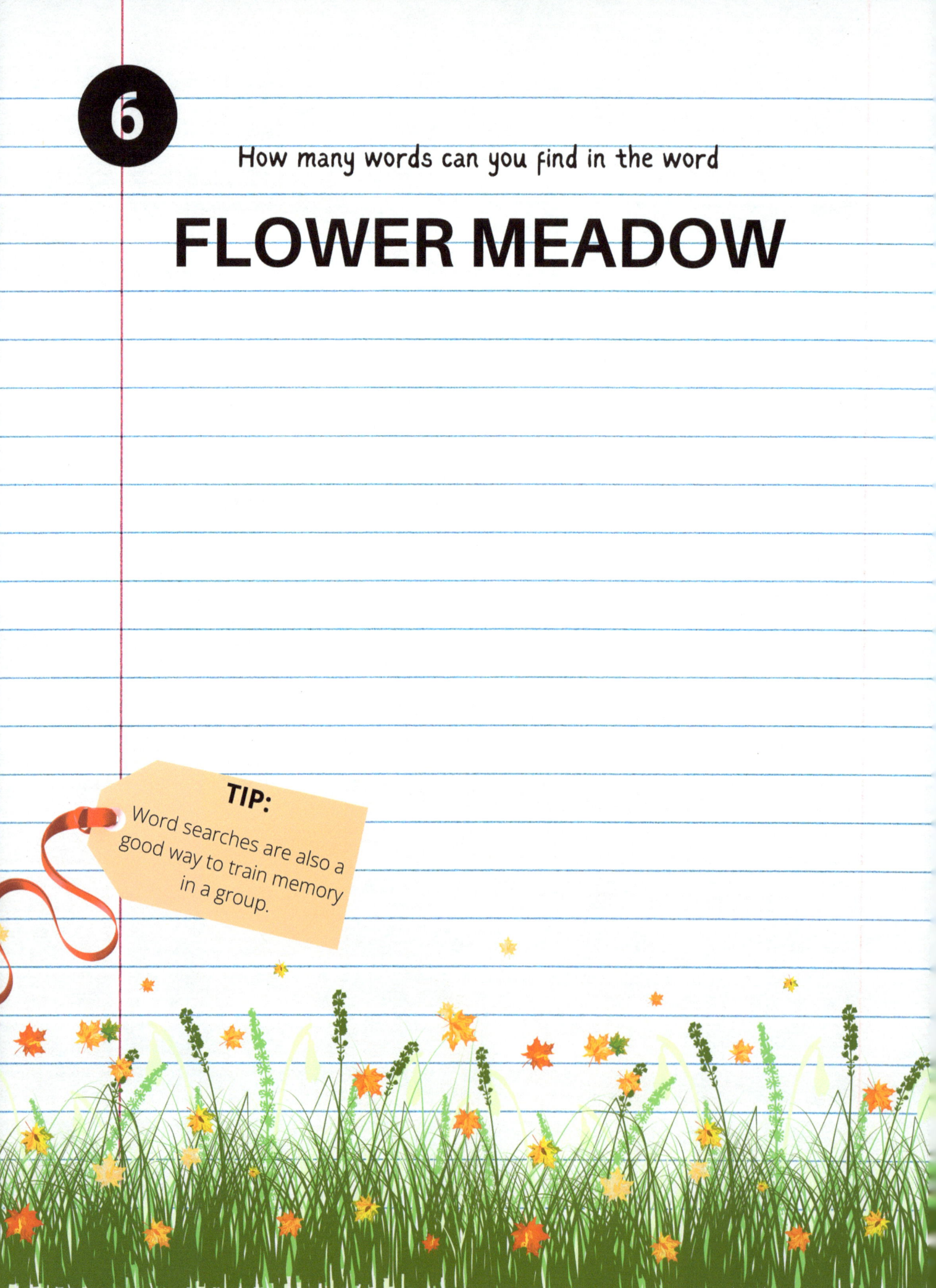

Snippets of memories

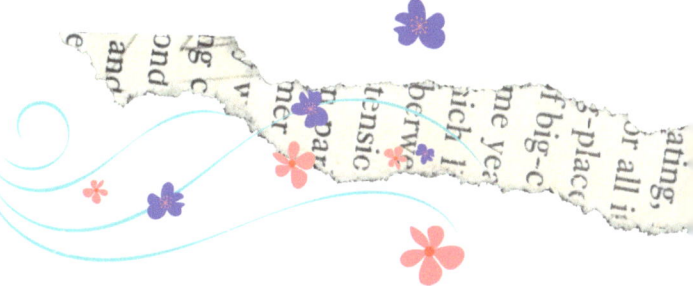

Remembering spring

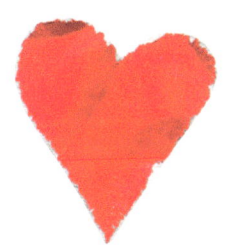

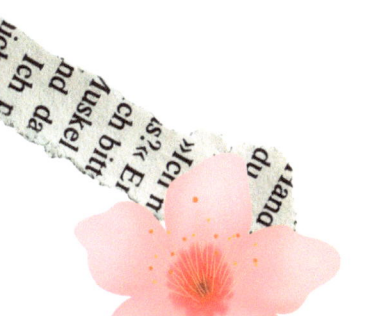

What did you like to do in spring?

Did you prepare the garden?

Have you been hiking or cycling?

Did you enjoy spring in nature?

What is your favorite spring memory?

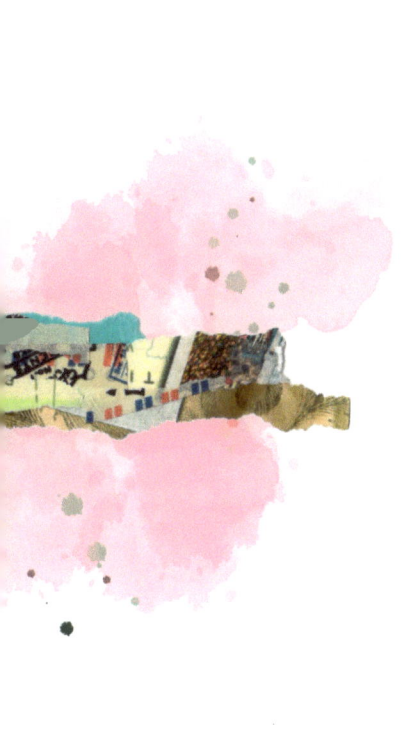

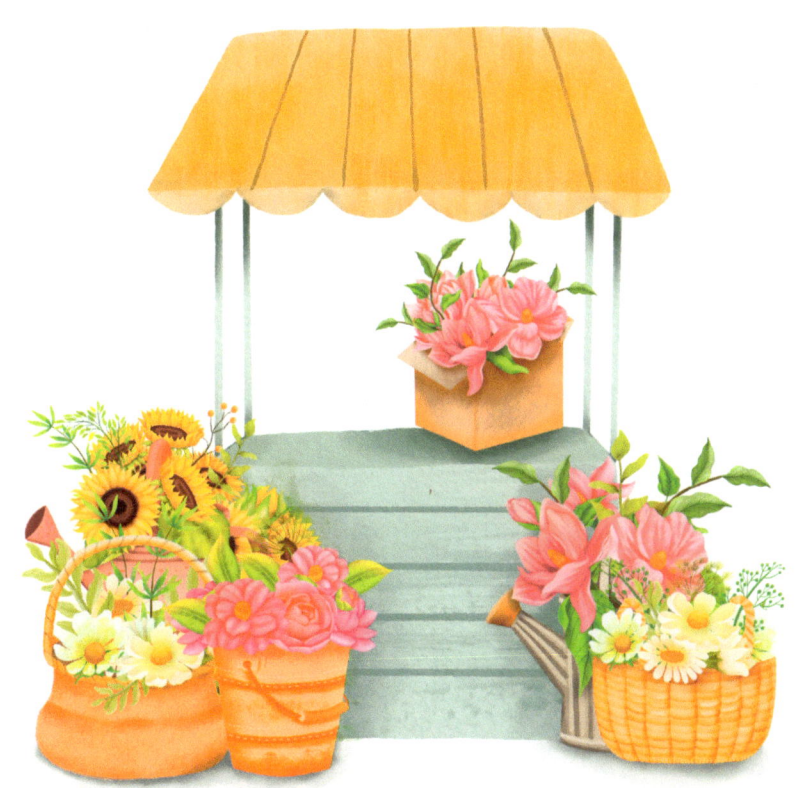

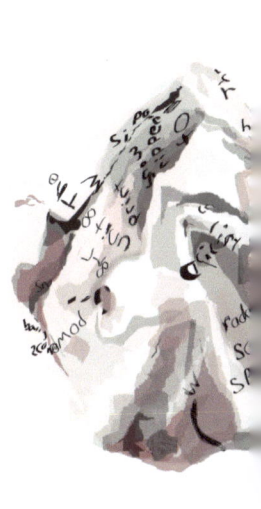

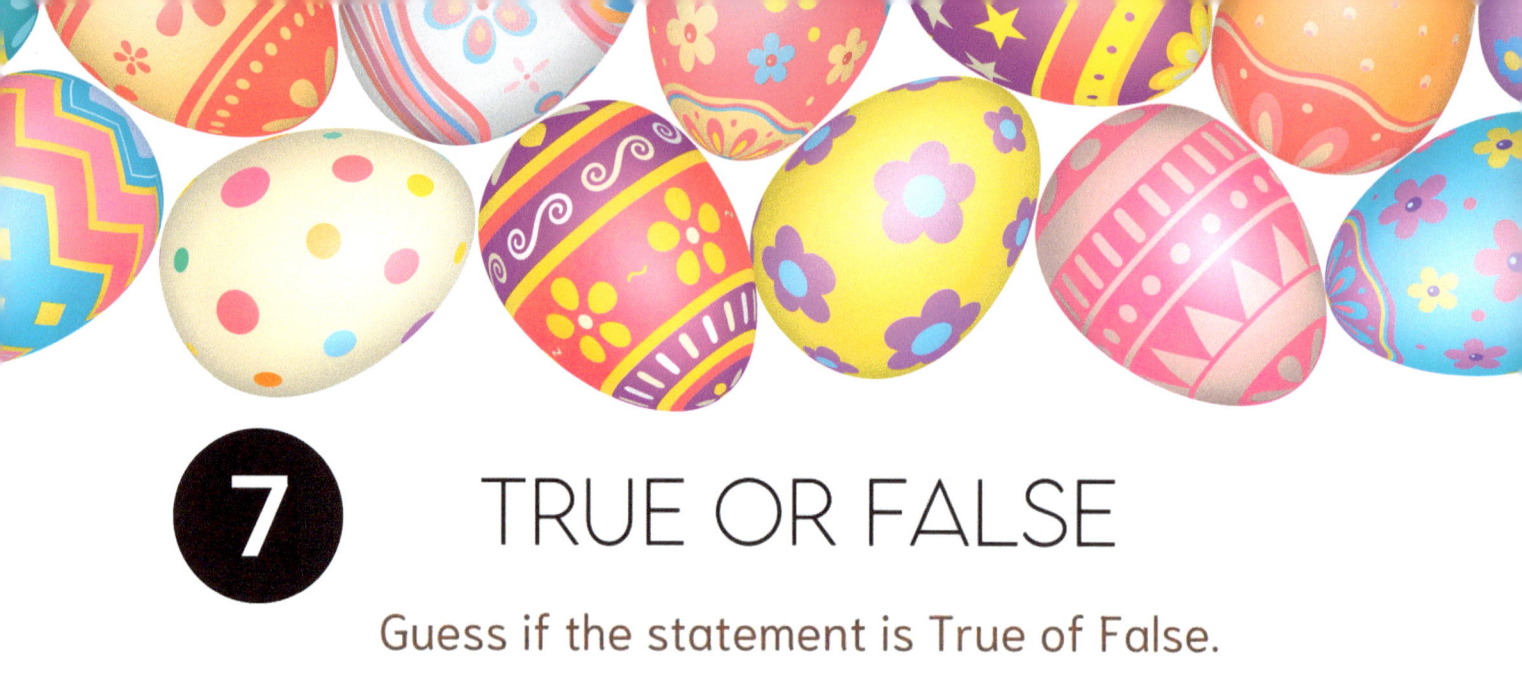

7 TRUE OR FALSE

Guess if the statement is True of False.

1. Judas betrayed Jesus for thirty gold coins? ....
2. The Easter Bunny legend originated in Germany? ....
3. In England, a rabbit is given as a traditional Easter gift. ....
4. Sweden has an Easter Wizard not an Easter Bunny. ....
5. Easter is named after the pagan goddess Ostara. ....
6. You shouldn't clean the house on Good Friday as per tradition as it brings bad luck. ....
7. Nick Easter is a former professional sportsman in baseball. ....
8. A rabbit named "Jumper" appeared in the Disney file Bambi ....
9. the rabbit in Alice in wonderland always carried a pocket watch with it. ....
10. around 90 million chocolate bunnies are produced each year. ....

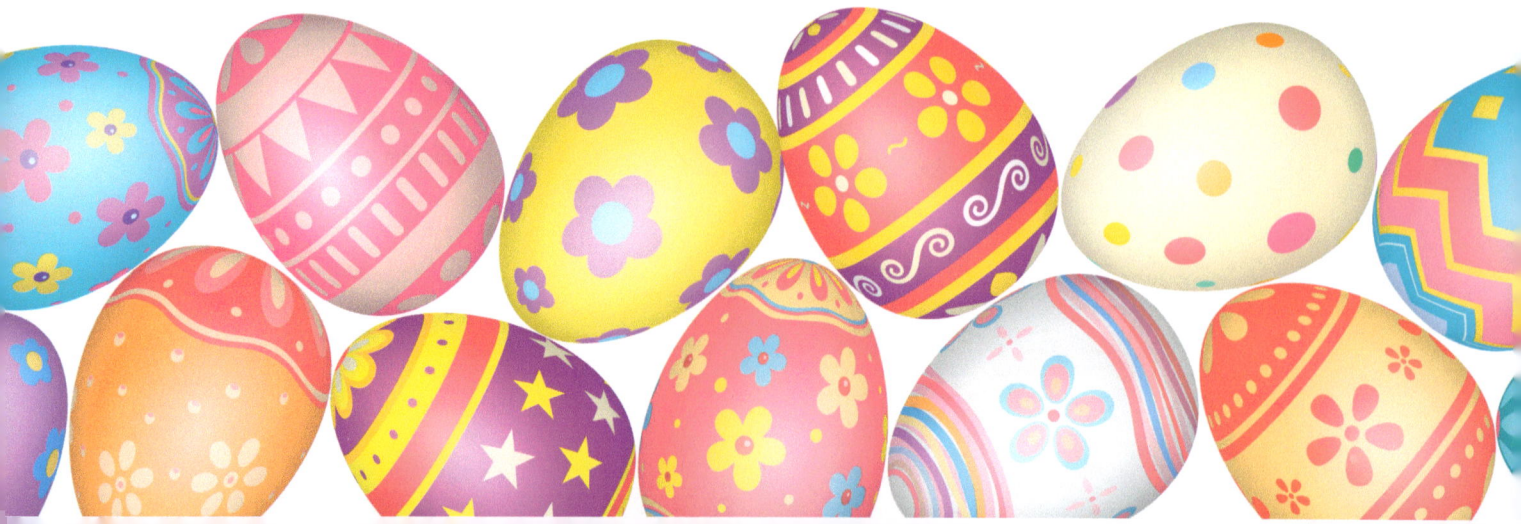

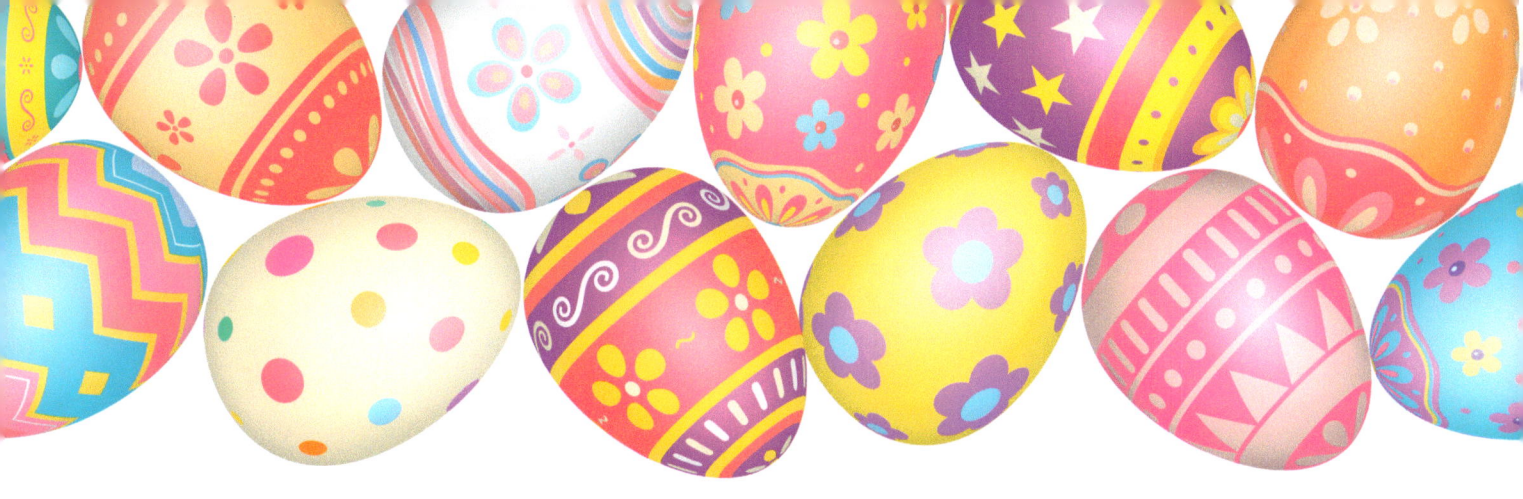

11. The largest Easter egg museum is located in Sweden. ....

12. The Sunday before Easter is called Palm Sunday. ....

13. Green is the most popular color among jelly beans. ....

14. Daisy flower is usually associated with Easter. ....

15. The Apostle Thomas doubted the resurrection of Jesus. ....

16. Fat Tuesday is the day before Lent. It is a time of overindulgence before fasting. ....

17. Lamb is also considered an Easter symbol besides bunny. ....

18. Tosca, Italy created the world's largest chocolate Easter egg. ....

Find the answers at the end of the book.

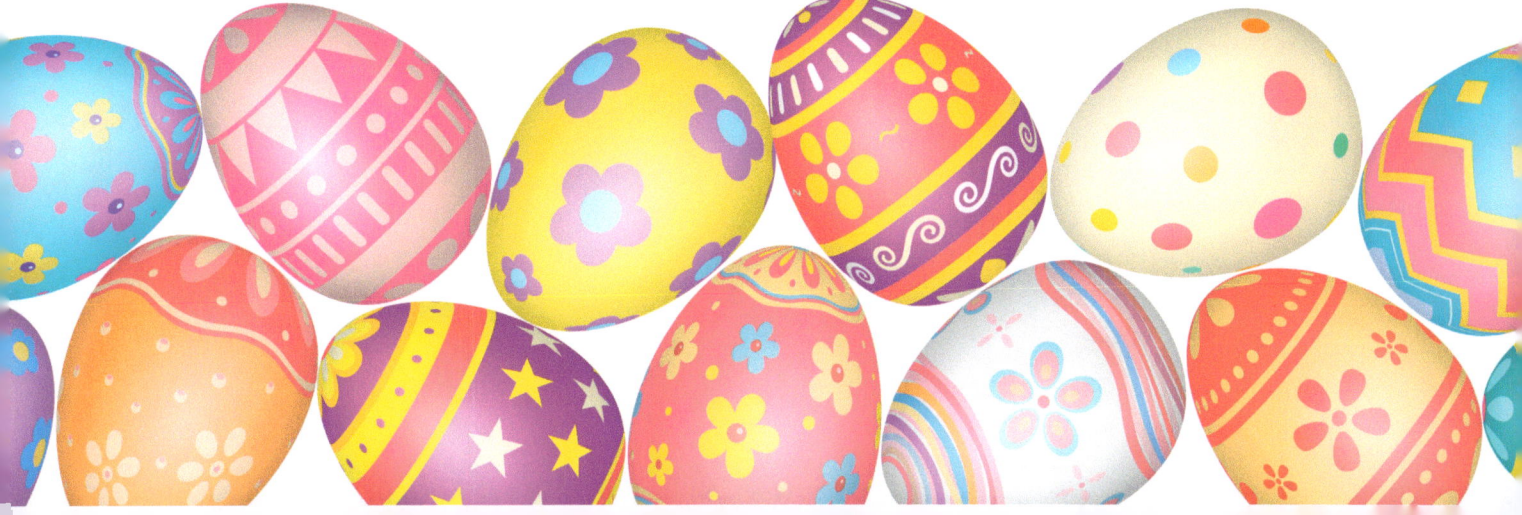

"A Light exists in Spring
Not present on the Year
At any other period –
When March is scarcely here

A Color stands abroad
On Solitary Fields
That Science cannot overtake
But Human Nature feels.

It waits upon the Lawn,
It shows the furthest Tree
Upon the furthest Slope you know
It almost speaks to you.

Then as Horizons step
Or Noons report away
Without the Formula of sound
It passes and we stay –

A quality of loss
Affecting our Content
As Trade had suddenly encroached
Upon a Sacrament."

Emily Dickinson

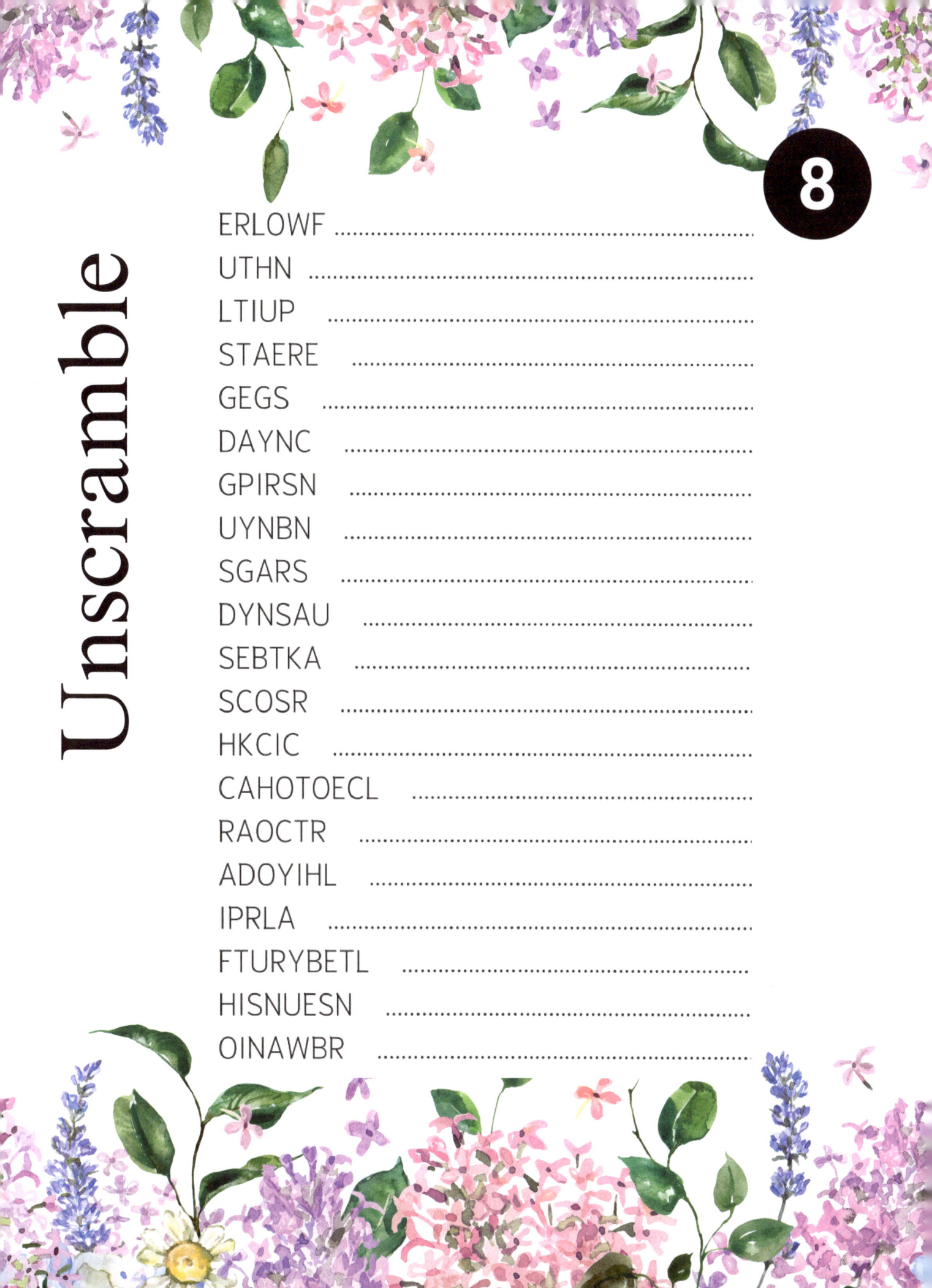

Unscramble

ERLOWF ....

UTHN ....

LTIUP ....

STAERE ....

GEGS ....

DAYNC ....

GPIRSN ....

UYNBN ....

SGARS ....

DYNSAU ....

SEBTKA ....

SCOSR ....

HKCIC ....

CAHOTOECL ....

RAOCTR ....

ADOYIHL ....

IPRLA ....

FTURYBETL ....

HISNUESN ....

OINAWBR ....

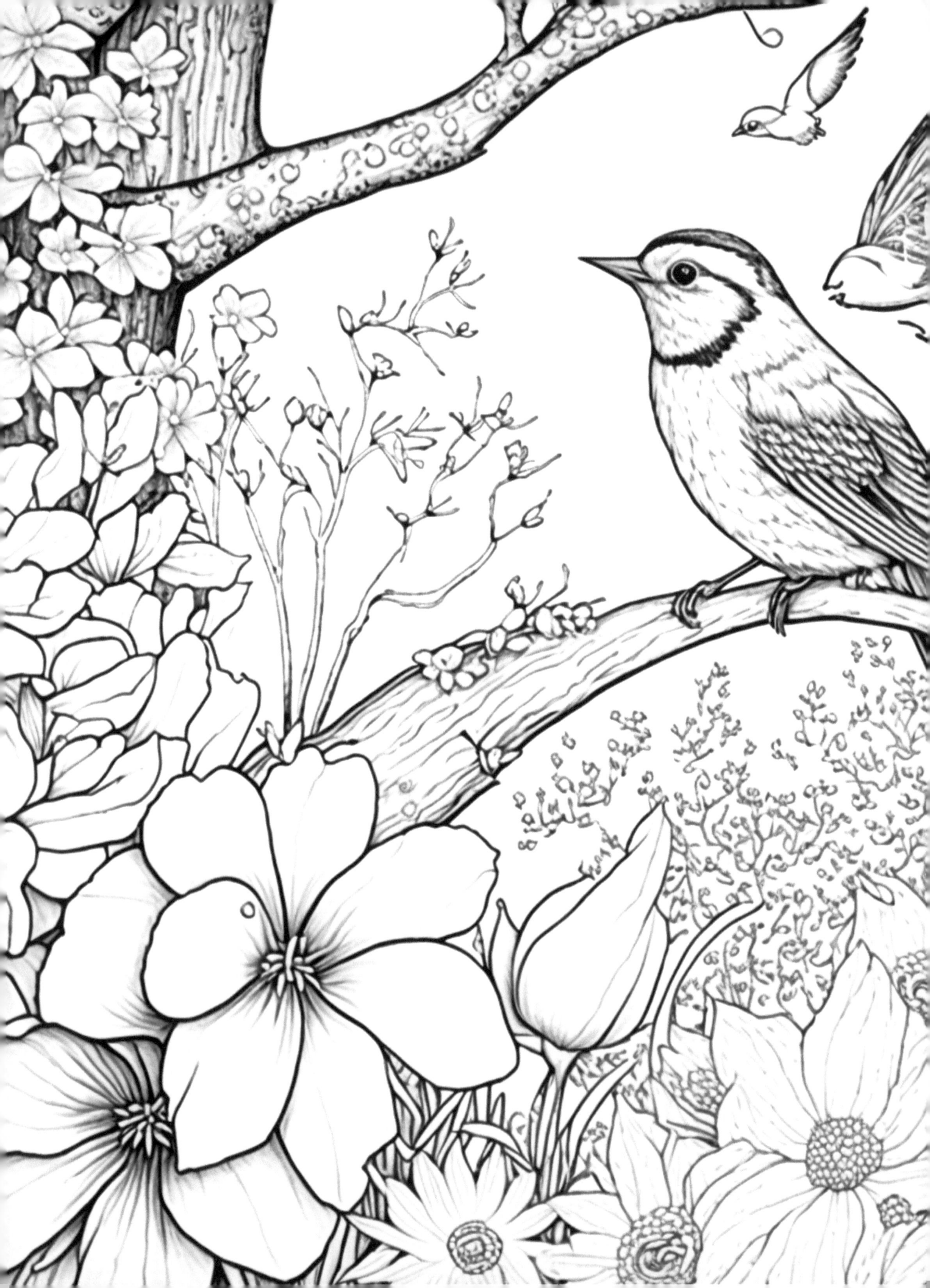

The bunny wants to go to
the Easter basket.
Find the way?

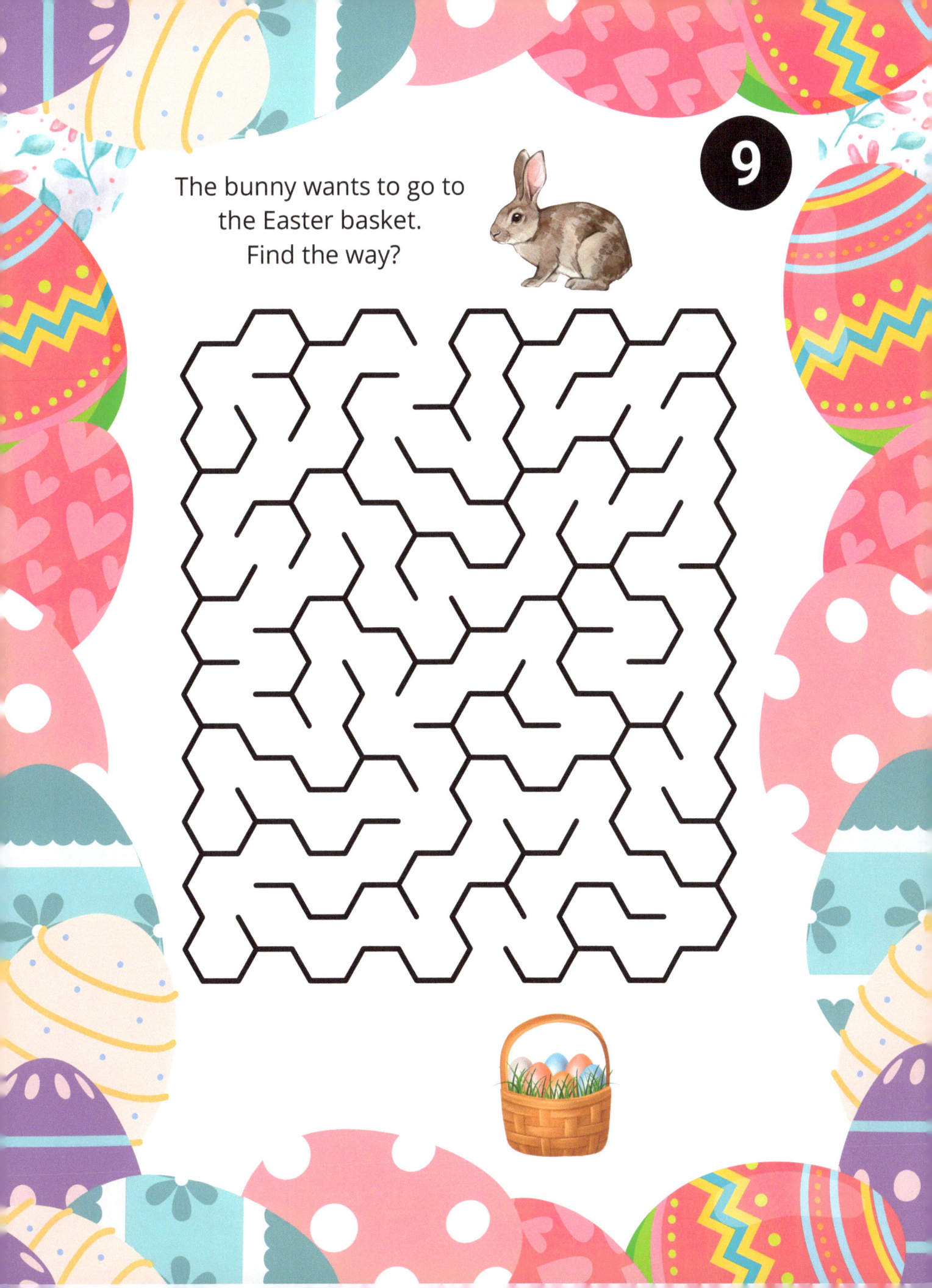

Herb time

When the first herbs grow again in spring, it's time for a delicious recipe with herbs, for example

Herb omelette

Ingredients:

2 Eggs
1 tablespoon milk
Butter to fry
1/4 cup chopped herbs
(e.g. parsley, chives, dill)
salt and pepper to taste

Preparation:
Whisk eggs and milk in a bowl and season with salt and pepper.
Melt butter in a pan over medium heat.
Add the chopped herbs to the pan and fry briefly.
Pour the egg mixture into the pan and let it set over medium heat for about 2-3 minutes.
Carefully turn the omelette over and fry on the other side for another 1-2 minutes.
Slide the omelette onto a plate and serve.

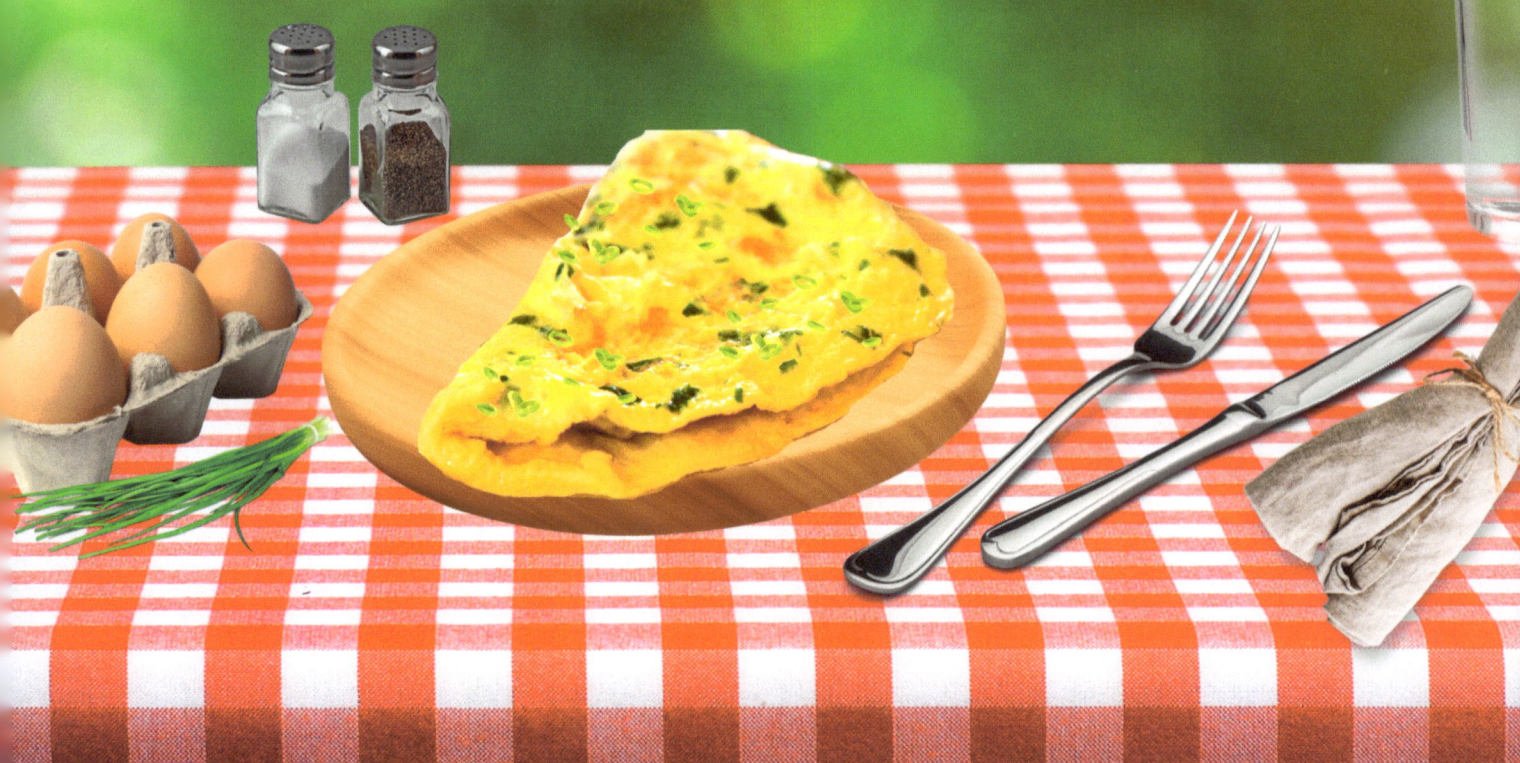

Hand-eye coordination

FIND YOUR WAY FROM ONE SIDE TO THE OTHER: TAKE YOUR TIME, TRY NOT TO TOUCH THE LINES

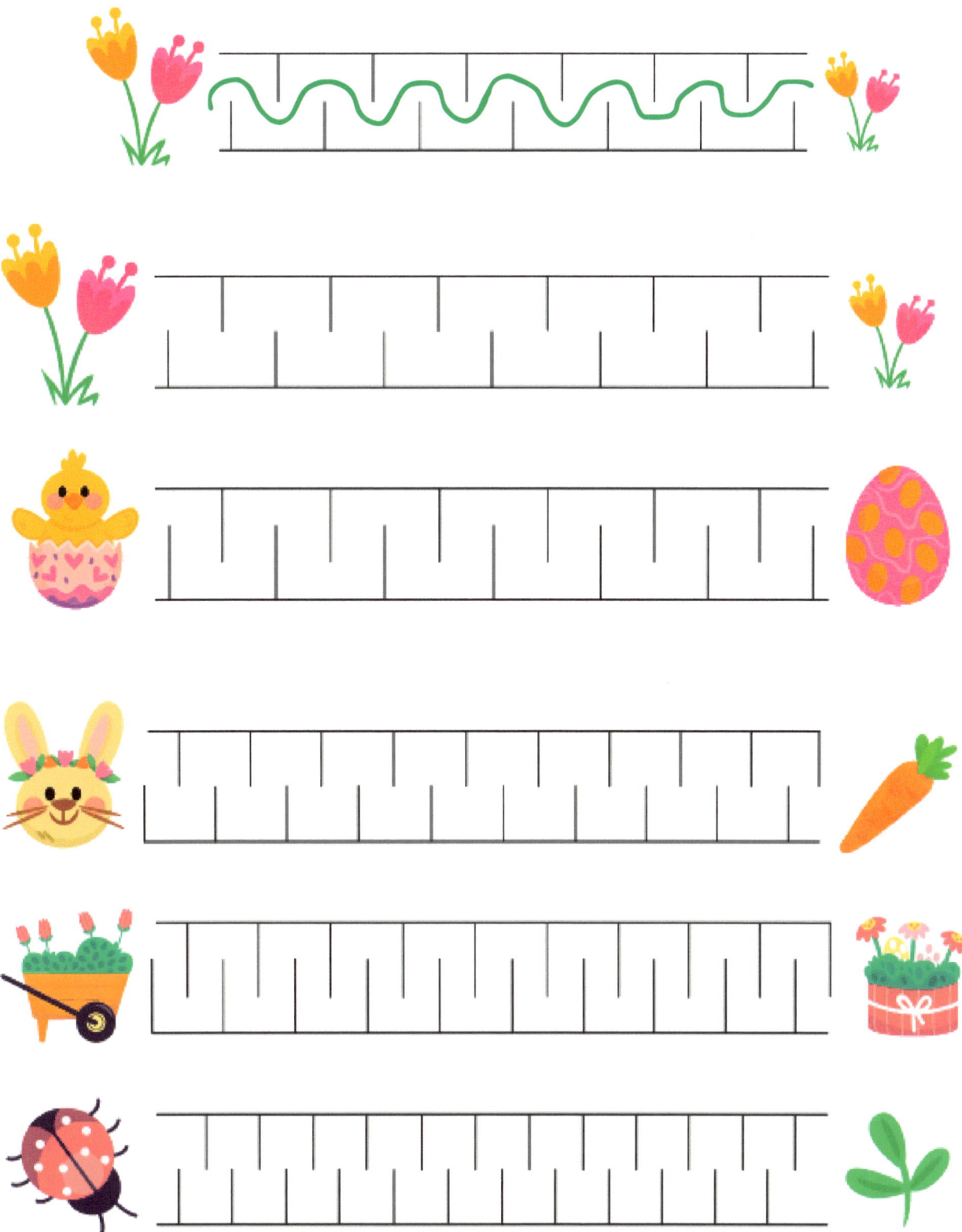

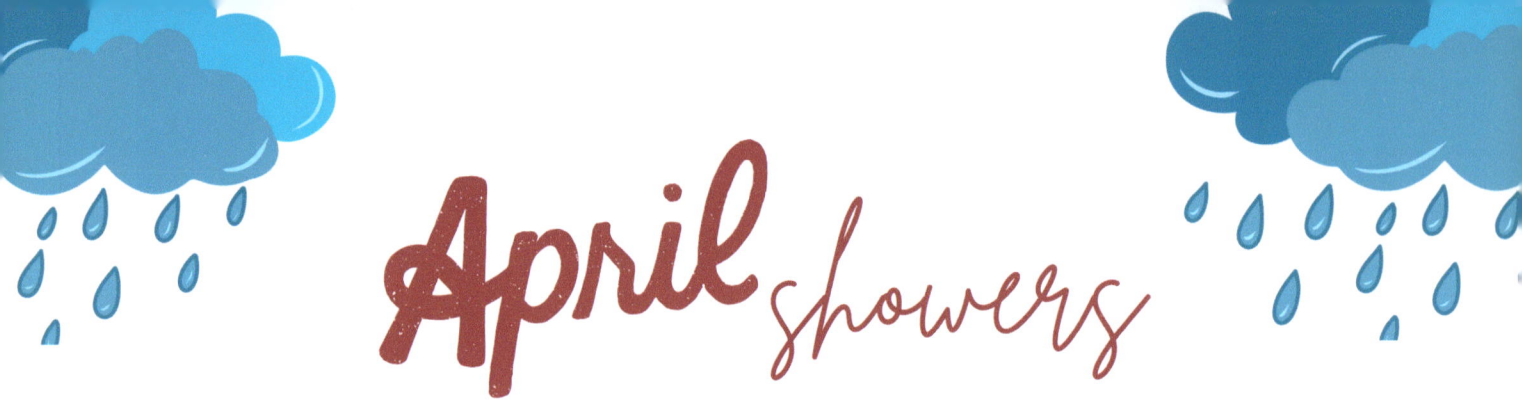

April showers

Verse 1
Life is not a highway strewn with flowers,
Still it holds a goodly share of bliss,
When the sun gives way to April showers,
Here is the point you should never miss.

Verse 2
Though April showers may come your way,
They bring the flowers that bloom in May,
So if it's raining have no regrets,
Because it isn't raining rain you know, it's raining violets.

Chorus
And where you see clouds upon the hills,
You soon will see crowds of daffodils,
So keep on looking for a <u>bluebird</u>,
And list'ning for his song,
Whenever April showers come along.

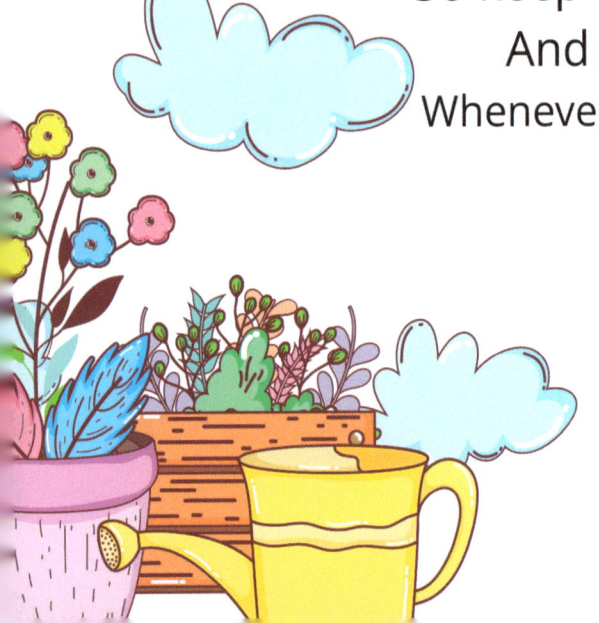

10 Do you know the spring flowers?

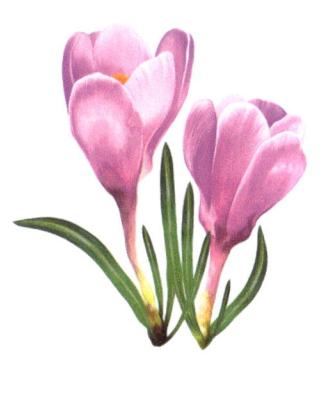

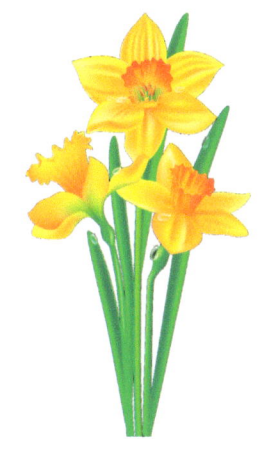

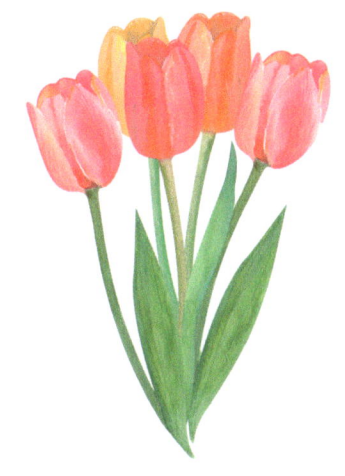

....

....

....

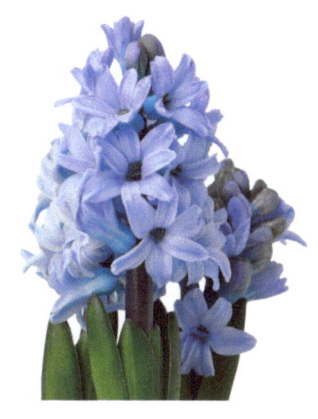

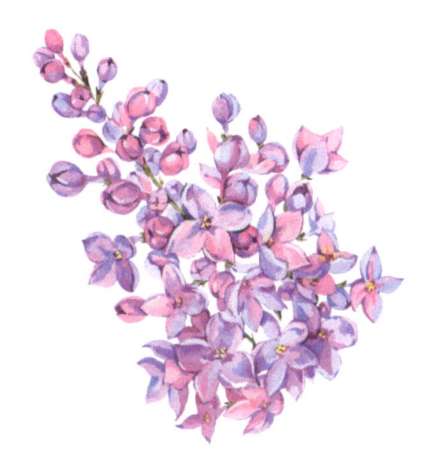

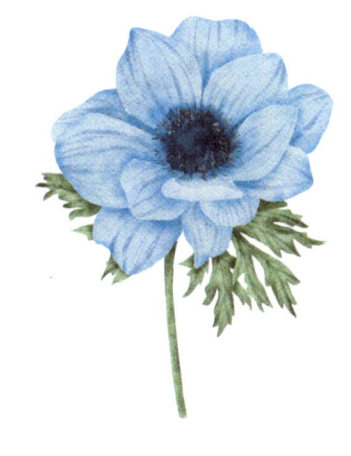

....

....

....

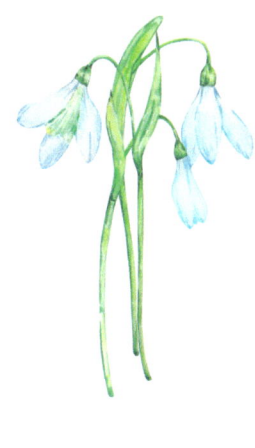

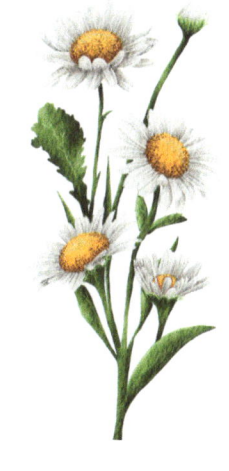

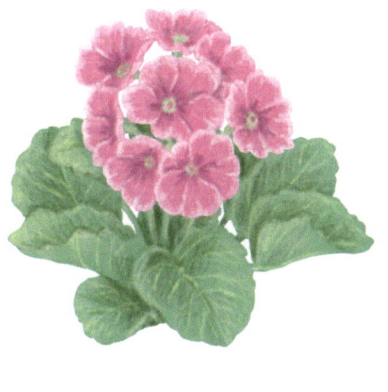

....

....

....

FACT OR FICTION

Answer Fact or Fiction for each statement.
Whoever gets the most correct wins!

.... Easter always falls between March 22 and April 25.

.... The second largest holiday for eating candy is Easter.

.... The rabbit is an ancient symbol of fertility

.... The cuckoo brings Easter eggs to children in Switzerland.

.... The lily represents "new life" or resurrection of Christ.

.... The tradition of the Easter bunny originate in England.

.... A kangaroo is use in Australia instead of Easter bunny.

.... Cadbury was found in Birmingham in 1824.

.... Easter island is part of Belgium.

.... The Sunday before Easter is called Palm Sunday.

.... Rabbits are considered rodents.

.... Rabbits cannot vomit.

.... Rabbits can live between eight to 12 years.

.... The rabbits constantly groom themselves.

COUNT AND CIRCLE THE CORRECT NUMBER

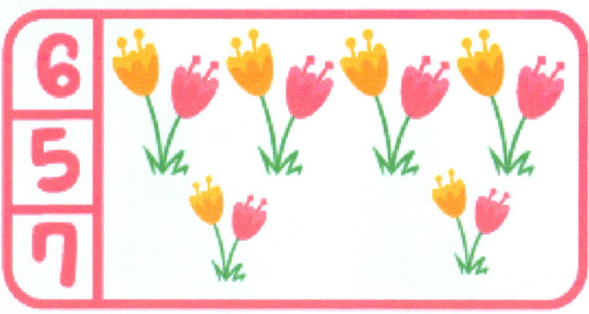

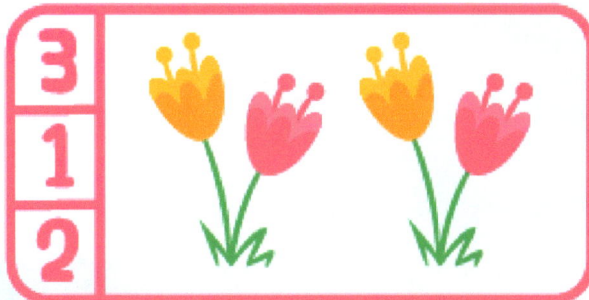

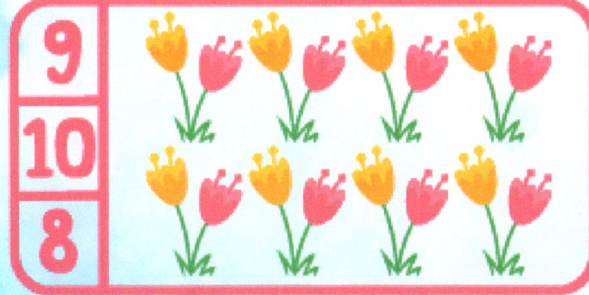

As a group activity make copies and see who is first.

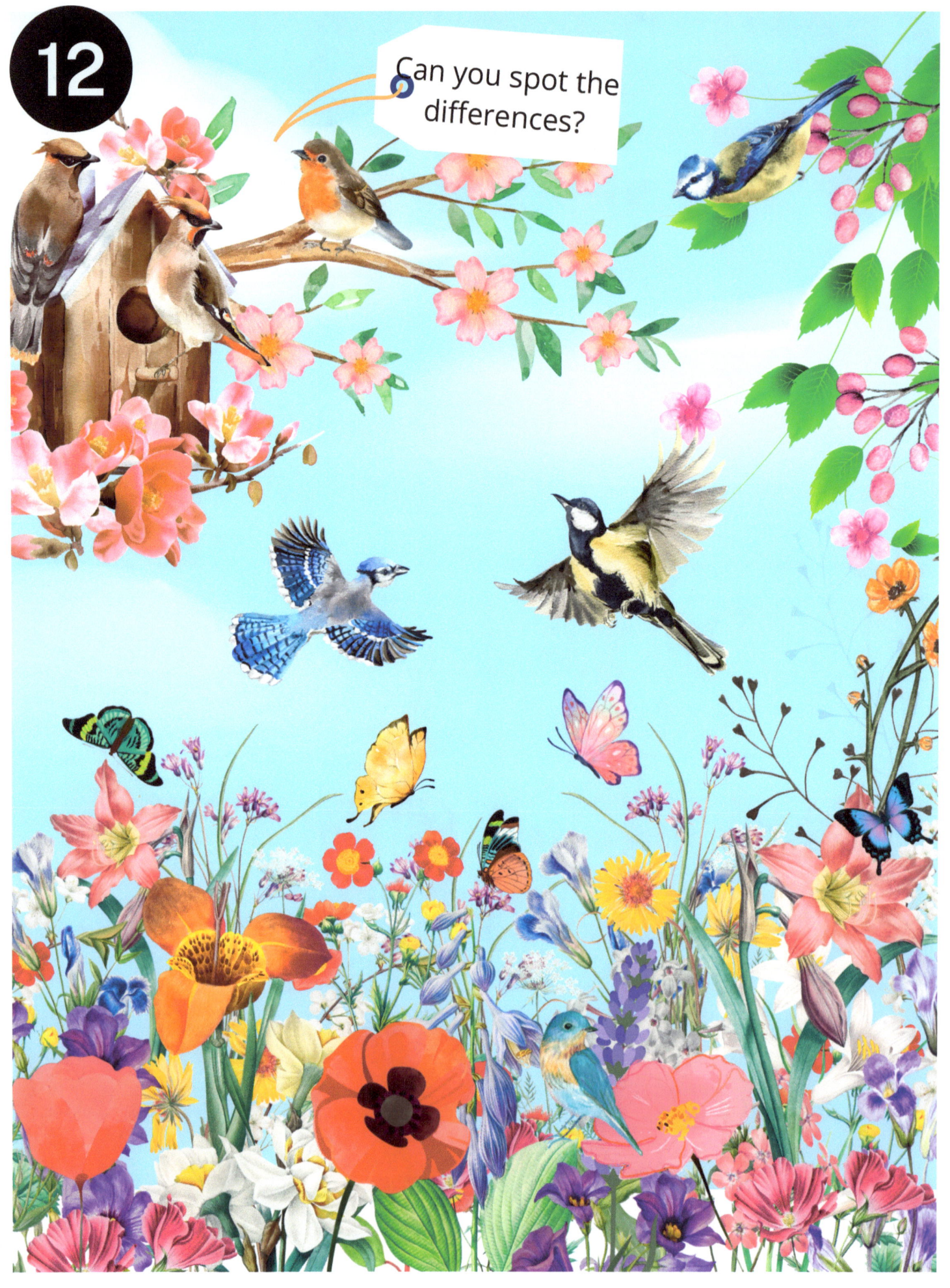

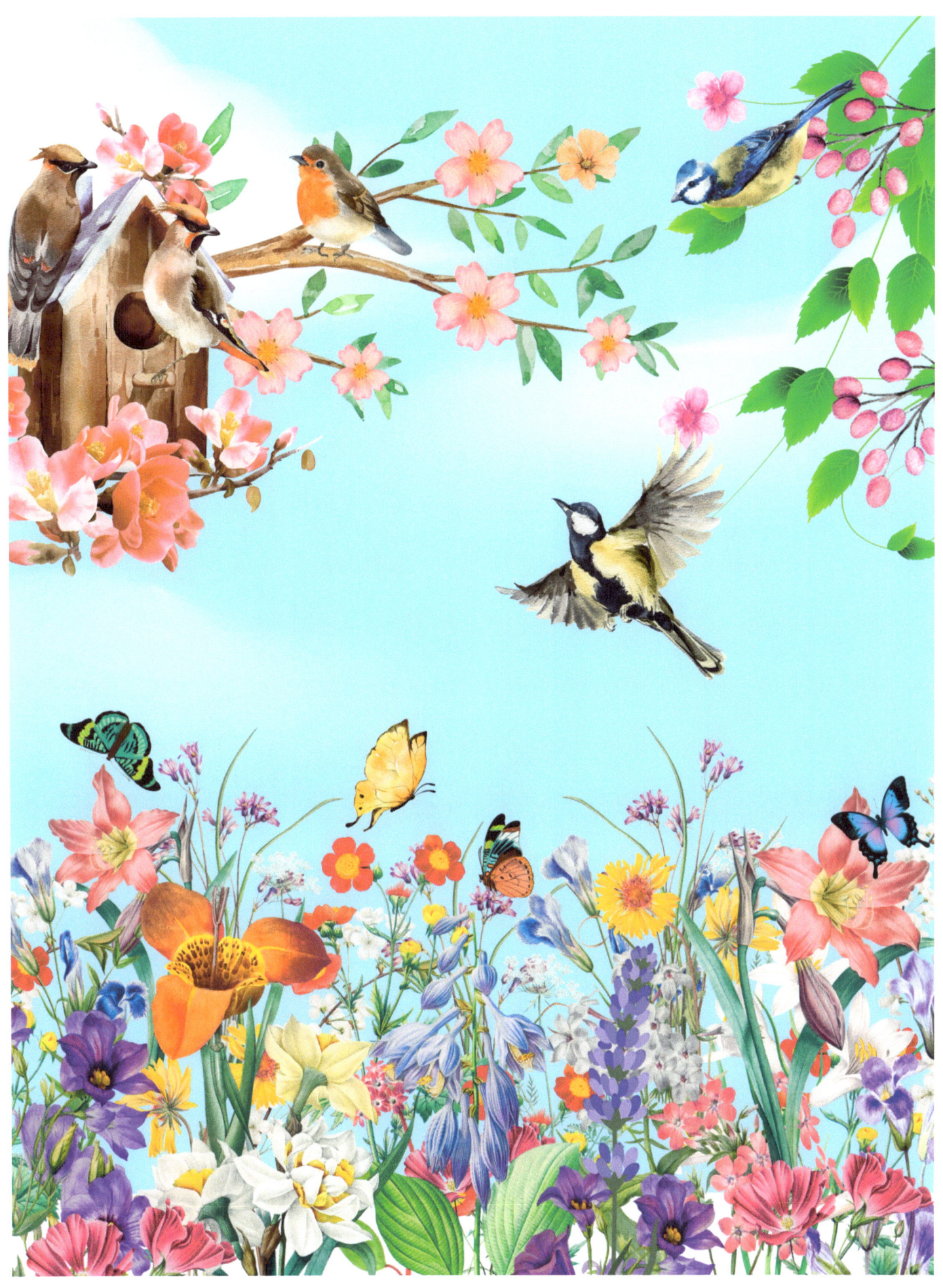

Count the different objects or animals in the picture and write the correct number in the boxes below

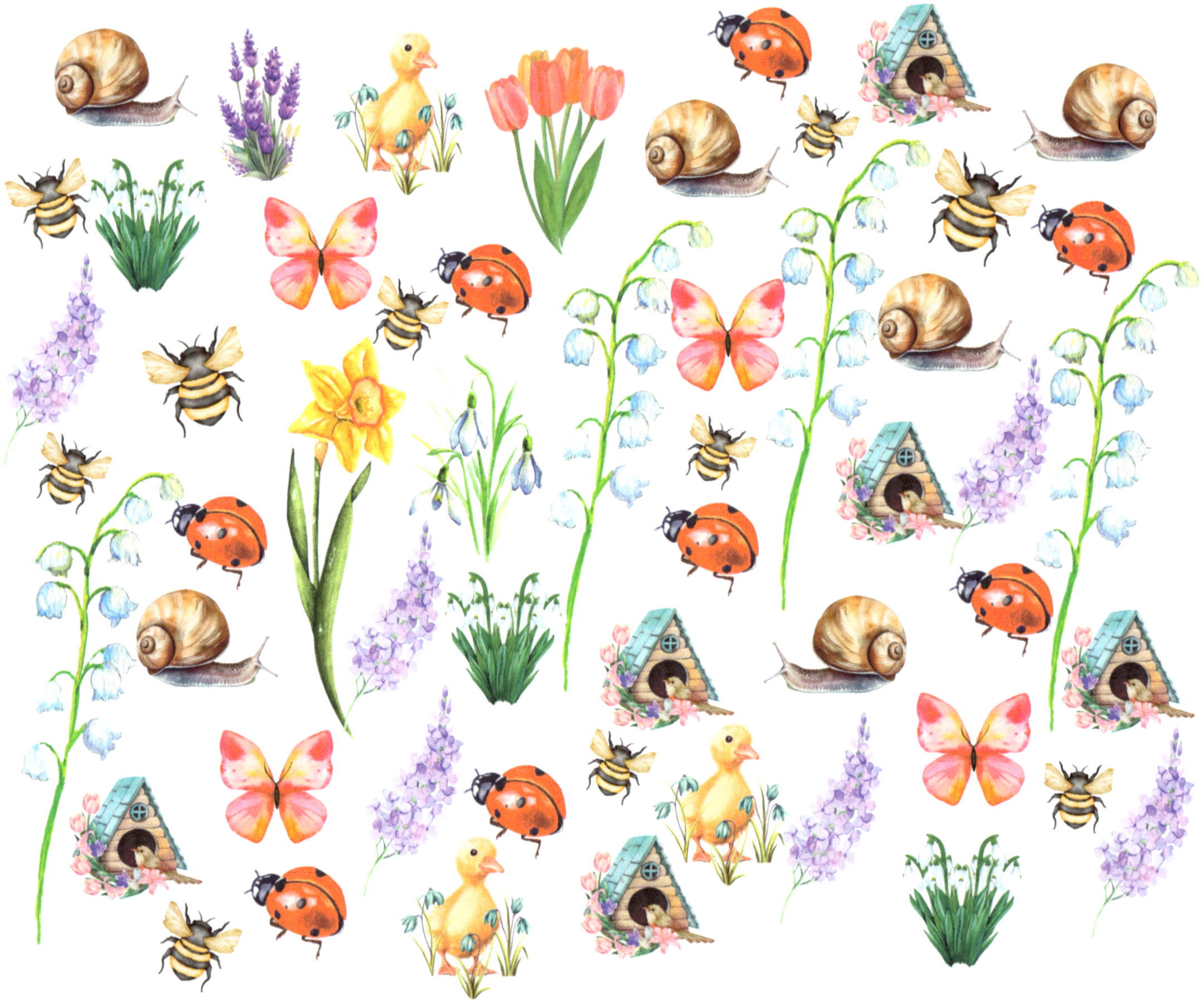

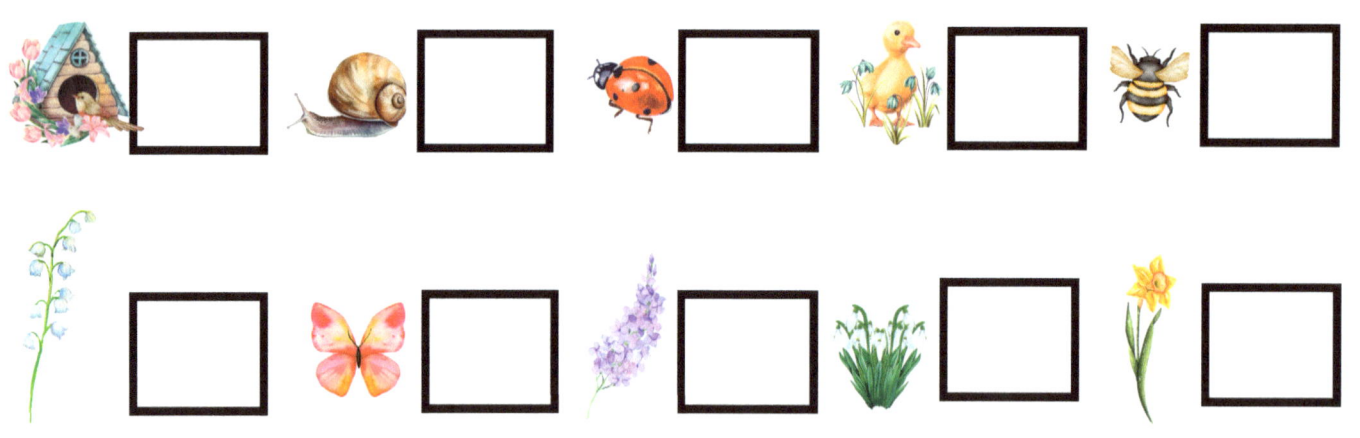

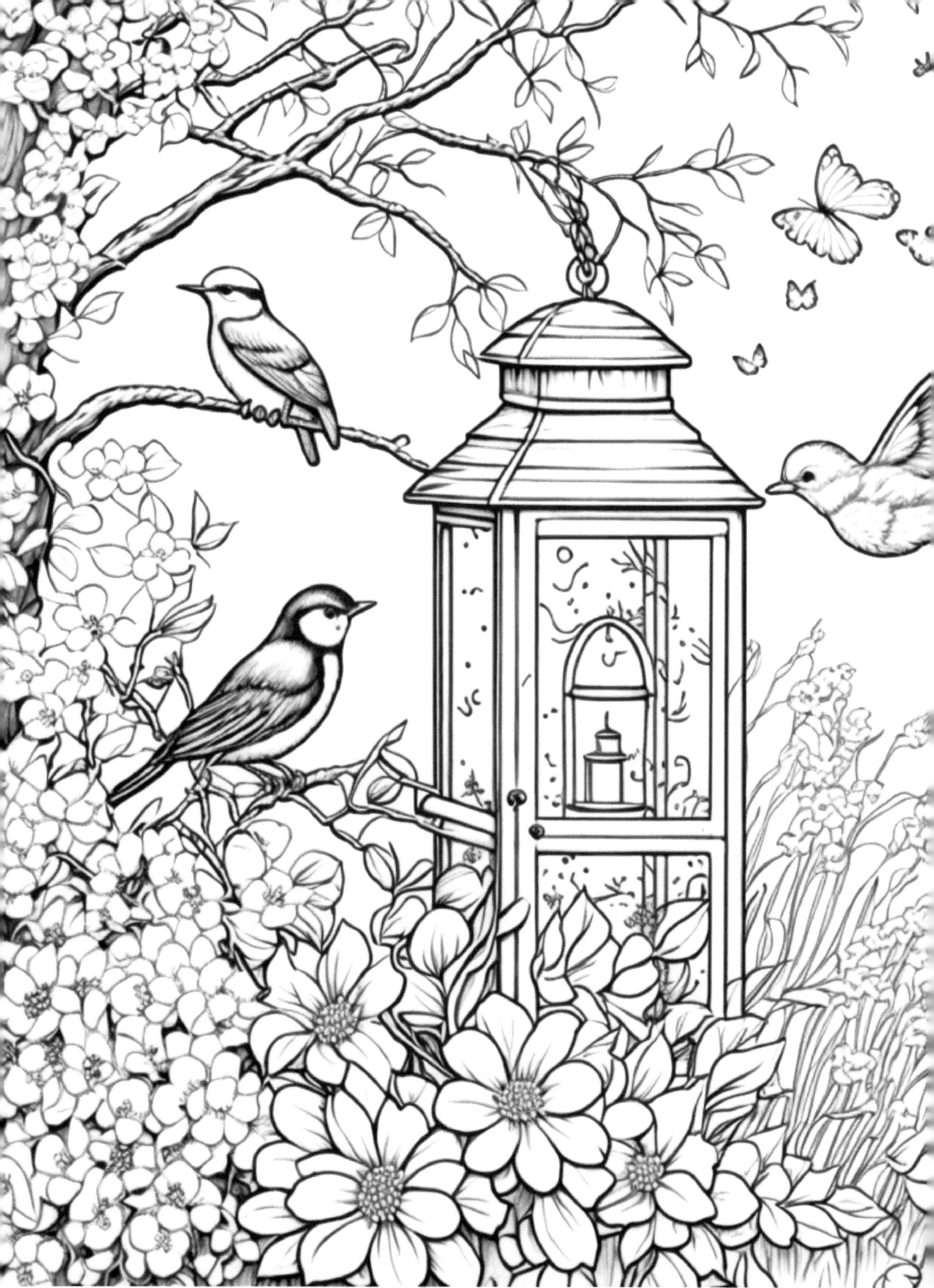

concentration

1. How many of each object can you find in the picture?
2. Write the number next to the illustration
3. It becomes easier if you give the objects colors.

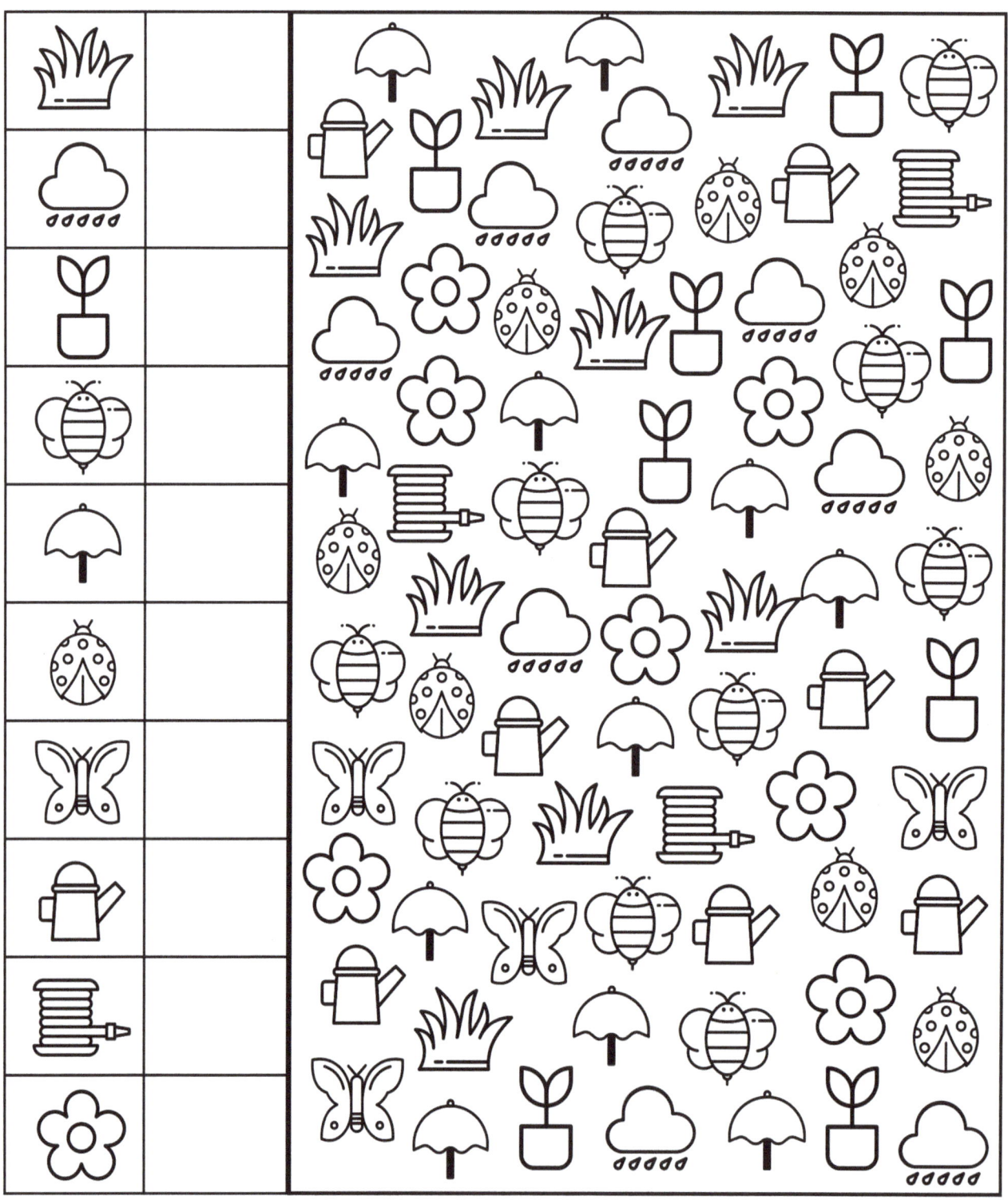

How do I use this book?

My books for activating seniors are suitable for both individual care and group lessons. - Get creative!

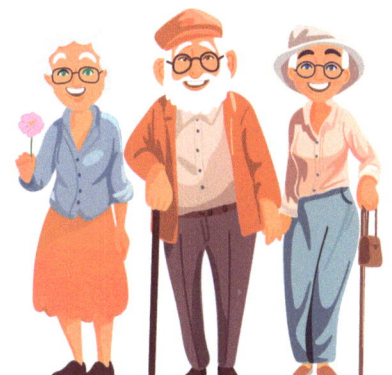

Why group activities?

Group activities for seniors offer numerous benefits, including:

Regular stimulation of the brain can maintain and improve cognitive abilities and prevent age-related impairments.

Social interaction: Group activities and games enable contact with other people, building new friendships and reducing loneliness. This significantly promotes mental health.

Seniors feel understood and accepted among their peers, which makes it easier for them to talk about their feelings and support each other. This makes it easier for them to deal with emotional challenges and makes it easier for them to accept the changes that come with age.
Group activities can improve physical health and reduce the risk of falls.

How do I use this book for group activities?

Ball games: Use a ball to solve various puzzles in the book together. For example with ABC lists on various topics. Say the letter and throw or pass the ball to a teammate who says a term with that first letter. The teammate gives or throws the ball to another teammate as a sign that he or she will continue. Stay with a letter until no one can think of a word for it and then move on to the next letter. Or go through them in order.

TIP: In my experience, it is easier to stay on a letter for longer, as people with (incipient) dementia sometimes need a little longer to think of a term. And be lenient, sometimes other players say words that don't start with that letter but contain that letter, that's ok too. Praise the effort and not the result.

The ball game can also be used well for all of the biographical questions in the book. This means everyone can contribute to a topic.

Artistic Creativity:

Activations that promote artistic creativity are great opportunities for a sense of achievement, socializing and increasing self-confidence.

Use the coloring pages (copies) to color together.

You can create small group lessons using the painting and craft instructions. The instructions are always designed in such a way that with a little support everyone can achieve a result. It's not about perfect implementation, it's about having fun doing things together.

Set up a place where the finished pictures can be displayed, picture frames or a pin board. Or decorate your living area with the pictures. Especially when resources are dwindling, the fact of having created something is very important and promotes self-confidence.

Singing, poetry and reading:

Singing together is always popular, so you will find songs, poems or stories on the respective topic in every book.

Put together a group and create a sociable atmosphere using various elements of the book. Introduce the topic. Start with a song or biographical questions (memory snippets), then read a poem, for example. The songs and poems are selected so that older people often know them from their youth. This is how memories are awakened. Give the group space to talk and exchange ideas. You will be surprised how many contributions come naturally once memories have been awakened through biographical impulses such as songs and poems.

Entertaining guessing games are great fun in a group and create a feeling of community.

Solve puzzles such as picture crosswords, mirror writing puzzles, search pictures, puzzle questions or proverb puzzles together. If necessary, make copies of this. For fitter residents, you can also turn it into a competition, for example: Who can find all the differences in the search picture first?

But be careful: avoid frustration for weaker players, help here or put the group of players together so that the group is homogeneous.

Bingo, board and dice games

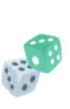
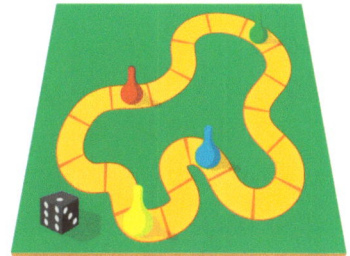

are also ideal for group lessons, stay relaxed and informal here.

People with dementia sometimes have difficulty with the rules of the game. Be generous here. Inverted numbers in bingo do happen. Here too, praise the effort and recognition of individual numbers. For some people this is a big achievement.

Don't say: "No, the number is wrong" but try to help diplomatically and possibly control it. The focus is always on having fun and not on the perfect result.

The same applies here: the more homogeneous the group, the less pressure there is for weaker players.

Maybe there will be the possibility of having several small rounds of games for fitter and weaker residents.

Enjoy together:

Seasonal recipe ideas invite you to cook and enjoy together. Of course they are just a suggestion. Your residents can probably think of many other recipes.

See what can be implemented in your area. Who else can actively help and wants to? Even those who only participate verbally, sniff or watch are actively involved! Everyone participates according to their ability.

Some people are just eating together, and that's okay too.

Smells while cooking or baking, feeling different textures or foods, and visually witnessing how a meal is prepared bring back many memories and promote a sense of togetherness in the group.

Of course, compliance with hygiene regulations is a given. Hand washing, disinfecting, rubber gloves and a clean work area are basic requirements for shared cooking activities.

Always include a few more foods that you can touch, feel and smell and that are not used for consumption.

This way you can stimulate all your senses and be on the safe side when it comes to hygiene.

Note:

When it comes to group activities with seniors, you have to keep in mind that the limitations in mobility and cognitive fitness are very different. It is therefore advisable to carry out different programs for different groups or to use the lowest level as a basis and then offer additional exercises for more advanced people.

Playful activities should also not be stressful for seniors if, for example, they are unable to do something due to motoric limitations. After all, playing should be relaxing and have a positive effect. Therefore, plan with enough breaks and do not overuse the time frame so that no one gets tired.

Individual care - beautiful moments for two.

All content is of course also suitable for individual support or self-employment. They can best assess what their resident, the person being cared for or their relative can still do or where help is needed.

Use the content for biographical conversations, look at the pictures together, read or sing together.

Solve the puzzles together; in a two-person situation, you can provide just as much support as is necessary.

Many elements are also suitable for self-employment.
Anyone who can still read or solve puzzles themselves can work through the book at their own pace and keep their memory sharp.

Finally:

My books are based on my experiences working with seniors and people with dementia. I also write and design the books together with my facility residents, taking their wishes and ideas into account. When motor and cognitive skills become weaker, I see and experience how I can prepare classic content so that even weak residents can enjoy it. I often experience relatives bringing "preschool books" with them when their parents or grandparents have poor eyesight or have motoric problems. But people with dementia also see very clearly that these books or notebooks are made for children. I have often heard the sentence: "Look, they brought this to me, I'm not a child."

This gave rise to my idea of combining books with classic, well-known content, puzzles and games in large print, songs and texts into books that are based on the experiences and lives of adults.

The simpler and larger design and the rich illustrations that awaken memories make it possible for the content to reach people who have already degraded more.

I also notice again and again that books strengthen and make communication between generations easier.

Grandparents can also do a lot of content with their grandchildren or children.

I hope you also enjoy it together with your residents or relatives.

If you have any further ideas or wishes, please don't hesitate to write to me.
You can reach me at:

info@sogehtsmirgut.de

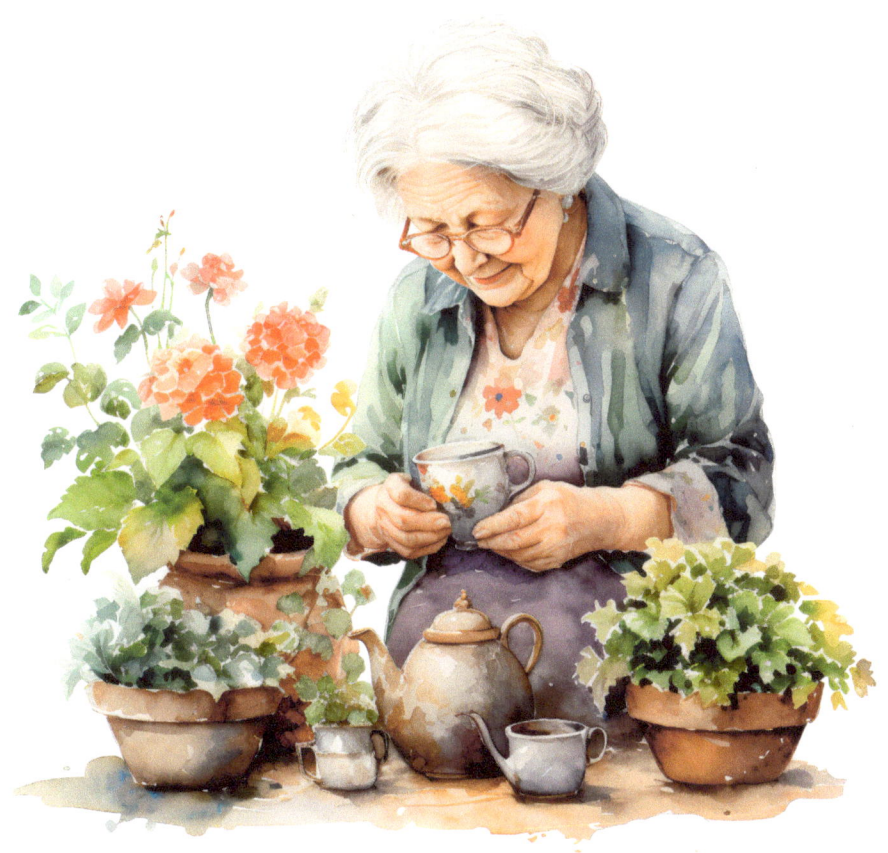

1 Mirror Mirror

TULIPS

SNOWDROP

HEYDAY

BUTTERFLY

NARCISSUS

PRIMROSES

BLOOMING

2 *Spring* WORD SEARCH

F	L	C	H	B	C	T	T	S	T	B	A	R	H
F	L	O	W	E	R	S	T	S	P	R	I	N	G
T	O	L	L	E	O	U	L	G	W	G	D	L	R
U	N	O	M	S	C	N	N	R	A	M	C	L	L
L	N	R	A	B	U	T	T	E	R	F	L	Y	I
I	I	S	Y	O	S	C	R	E	M	N	O	N	G
P	N	Ä	X	K	S	N	E	N	T	V	V	M	H
S	S	R	I	B	E	T	I	T	H	R	E	A	T
F	B	L	O	S	S	O	M	S	P	T	T	R	H
P	I	S	U	N	S	H	I	N	E	S	C	C	T
F	A	A	P	R	I	L	C	N	N	N	N	H	M

3

TRIVIA

Test your EASTER knowledge. Most correct answer wins!

1. What color was the first Easter eggs dyed?
   A. Blue   B. Yellow   **C. Red**

2. What flower is considered an Easter symbol?
   A. Lily   B. Tulip   C. Daisy

3. Easter is commemorated as the day that Jesus was:
   A. Born   **B. Resurrected**   C. Baptized

4. Where is the largest Easter egg museum in the world?
   A. Germany   **B. Ukraine**   C. Sweden

5. What country did the Easter Bunny tradition originate?
   A. Germany   B. Poland   C. France

6. What do white Easter Lilies represent?
   A. Optimism   B. wisdom   **C. Purity**

7. What is the date of Easter determined by?
   A. Weather   **B. The moon**   C. Date of the month

8. What egg-shaped candy is illegal in the United States?
   A. Cadbury   **B. Kinder surprise**   C. Robin eggs

9. What kind of meat is often associated with Easter?
   A. Lamb   B. Turkey   C. Pork

10. The most popular American Easter candy is:
    A. Peeps   B. Jelly Beans   **C. Cadbury egg**

Spring ABC

4

A – anemone, April
B – blooming, birds
C – countdown (counting down) to summer
D – Daisy
E – egg hunt
F – flowers
G – green grass
H – honeybees
I – Iris
J – jogging
K –
L – Ladybugs
M – May

N - Narcissus, nesting
O - outdoor activities
P - Picnic
Q - quacking
R - Rainbow
S - sunshine
T - Tulips
U - umbrella
V - violet
W - walking, warm weather
X - Extra sunscreen
Y - Outdoor yoga
Z - zoo - nice to visit in spring

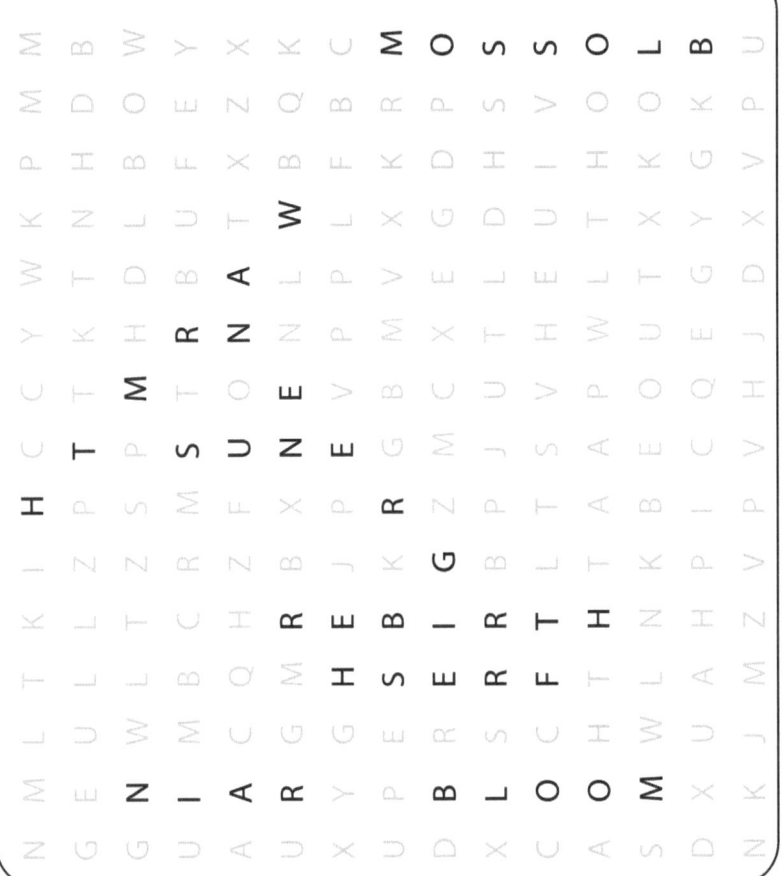

Word Bank

1. REBIRTH
2. SUN
3. WARMTH
4. FRESH
5. RAIN
6. BLOOM
7. GREEN
8. BLOSSOM

6 Flower Meadow

Some Words for example:

LOW, FLOW, FLOOR,
WOW, DEAR, WOOL, DOOR

How many did you find??

TRUE OR FALSE

Answer Key

1. Judas betrayed Jesus for thirty gold coins? .... FALSE
2. The Easter Bunny legend originated in Germany? .... TRUE
3. In England, a rabbit is given as a traditional Easter gift. .... FALSE
4. Sweden has an Easter Wizard not an Easter Bunny. .... TRUE
5. Easter is named after the pagan goddess Ostara. .... TRUE
6. You shouldn't clean the house on Good Friday as per tradition as it brings bad luck. .... FALSE
7. Nick Easter is a former professional sportsman in baseball. .... FALSE
8. A rabbit named "Jumper" appeared in the Disney file Bambi .... FALSE
9. the rabbit in Alice in wonderland always carried a pocket watch with it. .... TRUE
10. around 90 million chocolate bunnies are produced each year. .... TRUE
11. The largest Easter egg museum is located in Sweden. .... FALSE
12. The Sunday before Easter is called Palm Sunday. .... TRUE
13. Green is the most popular color among jelly beans. .... FALSE
14. Daisy flower is usually associated with Easter. .... FALSE
15. The Apostle Thomas doubted the resurrection of Jesus. .... TRUE
16. Fat Tuesday is the day before Lent. It is a time of overindulgence before fasting. .... TRUE
17. Lamb is also considered an Easter symbol besides bunny. .... TRUE
18. Tosca, Italy created the world's largest chocolate Easter egg. .... TRUE

ERLOWF .... FLOWER
UTHN .... HUNT
LTIUP .... TULIP
STAERE .... EASTER
GEGS .... EGGS
DAYNC .... CANDY
GPIRSN .... SPRING
UYNBN .... BUNNY
SGARS .... GRASS
DYNSAU .... SUNDAY
SEBTKA .... BASKET
SCOSR .... CROSS
HKCIC .... CHICK
CAHOTOECL .... CHOCOLATE
RAOCTR .... CARROT
ADOYIHL .... HOLIDAY
IPRLA .... APRIL
FTURYBETL .... BUTTERFLY
HISNUESN .... SUNSHINE
OINAWBR .... RAINBOW

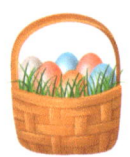

Der Hase möchte zum Osterkörbchen. Finden Sie den Weg?

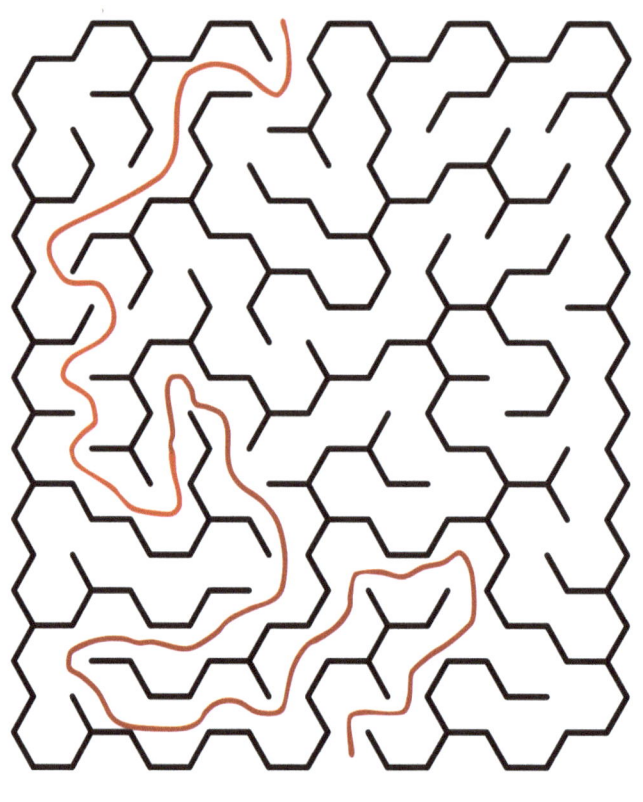

9

10

11

ANSWER KEY!

Fact	Easter always falls between March 22 and April 25.
Fact	The second largest holiday for eating candy is Easter.
Fact	The rabbit is an ancient symbol of fertility
Fact	The cuckoo brings Easter eggs to children in Switzerland.
Fiction	The lily represents "new life" or resurrection of Christ.
Fiction	The tradition of the Easter bunny originate in England.
Fiction	A kangaroo is use in Australia instead of Easter bunny.
Fact	Cadbury was found in Birmingham in 1824.
Fiction	Easter island is part of Belgium.
Fact	The Sunday before Easter is called Palm Sunday.
Fiction	Rabbits are considered rodents.
Fact	Rabbits cannot vomit.
Fact	Rabbits can live between 8 to 12 years.
Fact	The rabbits constantly groom themselves.

12

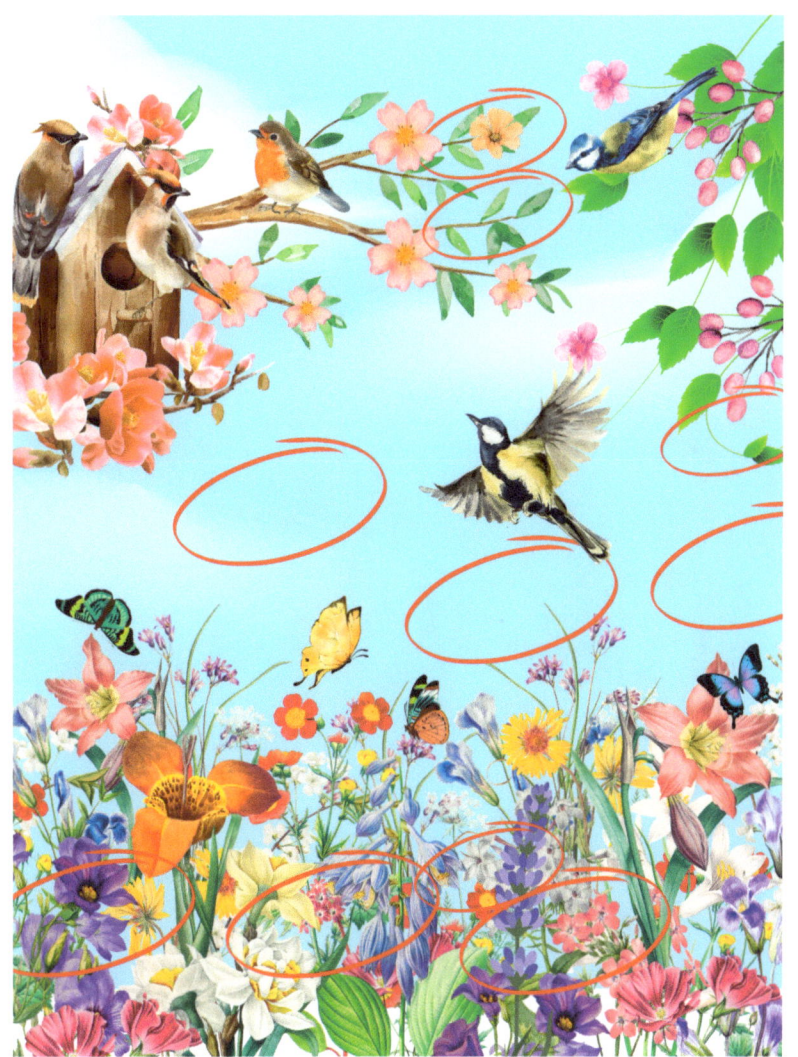

13

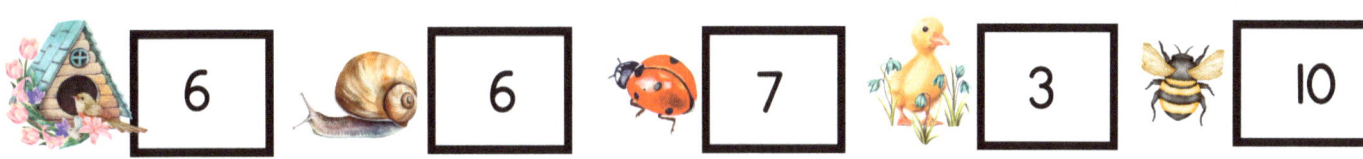

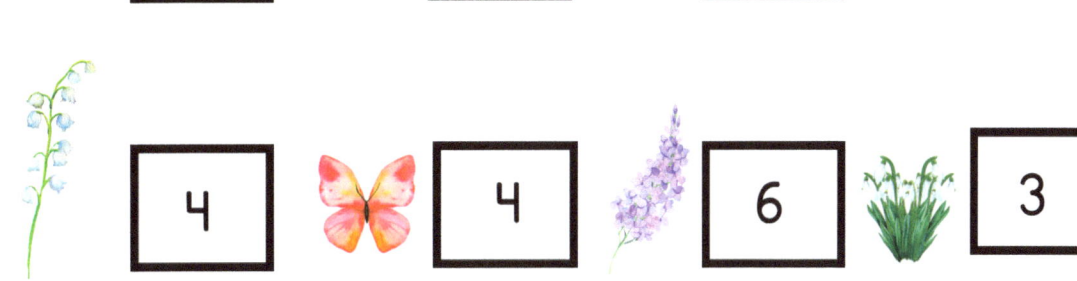